Dr Nowzaradan

Diet Plan Book

Lose Up to 30 Pounds in 4 Weeks with 1200 Calorie 30 Day Diet Plan and 100 Perfectly Portioned Recipes on a Budget - Suitable for Every Age.

Catharine Smith

Disclaimer

Table Of Contents

Part 1

Preface

CONGRATULATIONS It doesn't matter whether you choose a book on the topic of weight loss. It doesn't matter which book you choose out of the thousands of books available in the market, you have now decided that your weight should be a healthy weight and that is commendable. You value your time and you have decided that your precious time is not going to be wasted experimenting with techniques and looking for answers here and there to your problems and I tell you that you have come to the right place.

I value and respect the time and effort you are going to put into reading and practicing the book, and I promise you that you will get the return you desire. Every line in this book is written with a specific purpose in mind. The book sticks to its points and is as precise as possible without compromising the quality of the information and examples provided. This way you will get the information you need and get it quickly. At the end of each chapter the chapter summary is given in bullet points so that you don't have a problem with the book practice and you remember the important points.

Before you read the book I want to make you a promise that if you learn all the points and act upon them, you will come back from the book a different person with complete control over your time and a healthy weight.

Science Behind Dr. Now Diet

All animals and most species cannot choose their food as humans do because they do not have the freedom to choose. In simple terms, cows and buffaloes are attracted to grass by their inbuilt instincts. But humans does not have a fixed food instinct. He can choose food based on his judgment and this is against the theory of evolution.

Every culture and society worldwide has different food choices that are majorly different. So it is impossible to have one diet with the same suitable recipes worldwide. Animals have a stronger sense of food intake and dietary balance than humans which prevents them from overeating so animals eat to survive and that is why animals are not found overweight generally. When we are going through our infancy, we have an efficient food intake system that prevents us from overeating but as we grow older, our efficient system becomes inactive.

Diets have been popular for centuries. Each diet becomes popular for only two to three years, then a new diet replaces it and remains popular for two to three years. We try a diet to lose weight but it gets boring and when it gets boring we go back to our old habits so we gain the weight back.For long term weight loss we need to adopt healthy eating habits. We should practice chewing food 32 times.

Give twenty minutes to each meal. Do not watch TV and computer during meal time. Do not eat snacks between meals. Drinking a glass of water before each meal will make you feel fuller faster and ultimately reduce your calorie intake by eating less. Pay attention to the labeling of packaged foods. Remind Yourself of Serving Sizes Generally serving sizes aim to provide you with the right amount of food to eat and not to exceed more than one serving size.

Calorie content is more important and is often given in a serving size. For example, if the calorie content of a label is 160 calories per serving size and each package contains 8 serving sizes, the content will be 1280 calories.

Dr. Nowzaradan Diet Hidden Secret

The simple answer to the question of why we gain weight or why we gain more fat in our body is because carbohydrates make us so ; protein and fat do not. But if that's the case, we all know that people who are on a low-fat diet and lose weight are low-fat and relatively high in carbohydrates, so why shouldn't it be successful for all people?

When researchers tested the effectiveness of diets in clinical trials, they found that some high-fat diets actually lead to weight loss, which doesn't mean some of us gain fat because we eat carbs and then get lean again when we don't, but for others, avoiding fat is the answer? The simple answer is probably no.

A possible explanation for this is that any dieter that succeeds does so because the diet restricts fatty carbohydrates. Simply put, those who lose fat on a diet can do so because of what they're not eating- fattening carbohydrates not because of what they're eating. Whenever we go on any serious weight loss regimen we make some changes in what we eat in our diet.

In particular, we should avoid fatty carbohydrates because it is the easiest to eliminate and the most obvious one if we are trying to get in shape. First of all, drinking beer should be stopped, for example, or at least in moderation. We may think we are cutting calories but the calories we are cutting are carbohydrates and more importantly they are liquid pure carbohydrates with their fat content. Not to mention, fructose, which is particularly responsible for making soda sweet, is the same with fruit juices.

Replacing fruit juice with water is one of the easiest diet changes you can make, and you should get rid of candy bars, donuts and cinnamon buns. Again, understanding that we're cutting calories and maybe that's a way to lose fat, but we're also cutting carbohydrates, especially fructose.

You should replace starchy foods like potatoes, rice, bread, and refined foods like pasta with greens, salads, and whole grains. If we try to reduce a significant number of calories from our diet, we can also reduce the carbohydrates we consume. Even if your diet is to reduce fat calories, it is very difficult for you to reduce calories a day by reducing fat and therefore you should also eat less carbohydrates.

Low-fat diets that also reduce calories are as much or more low in carbohydrates. Simply put, when we try any conventional method and when it comes to 'eating healthy' we will remove the most fattening carbohydrates from the diet and some portion of total carbohydrates as well.

If you reduce the amount of refined carbohydrates in your diet, this will definitely help you lose body fat. Also when food products are made into low fat foods, the opposite happens. They remove some of the calories from the fat but then replace them with carbohydrates. In the case of low fat yogurt, for example, they remove most of the fat without replacing it with high fructose corn syrup. Instead of eating a fatty breakfast that will lead to weight loss, skipping carbs and leaving you satiated will make you fatter.

Doctor now say that it is very difficult to lose weight by just exercising. Rare are the people who start exercising to slim down but don't make any changes to what they eat. Instead, they cut back on their beer and soda consumption, cut down on their sweets, and maybe try replacing starches with green vegetables. Usually they do because they prevent something other than what we call fat. When calorie-restricted diets fail, as they usually do, it's because they restrict something other than the foods that make you fat.

The reason people go on a diet plan is because they restrict fats and proteins that don't have a long-term effect on insulin and fat storage but are needed for energy and cells and rebuilding them. They starve the entire body of nutrients and energy, or starve half of it instead of targeting fat tissue.

Any weight loss can only be sustained as long as the dieter can tolerate partial starvation, and even as the muscle cells try to obtain protein, the fat cells work to replace the fat they lose. Ultimately what we learn is that diet plans are only successful if we eliminate the fattening carbohydrates from the diet. Otherwise they will fail. What a diet plan should do is basically re-regulate fat so that it releases excess stored calories.

What Is Dr Now Diet ?

Doctor Nowzaradan has introduced a new rule in the diet plan world.

There are three aspects that affect our daily intake of calories. These three factors are what dr now refers to as the acronym F.A.T.

F stands for frequency, A stands for amount, and T stands for the type of food.

Frequency- The frequency of eating habits should be 2 or 3 meals a day. Do not have snacks in between meals.

Amount- The amount limits our calorie intake per day to 1200 calories, and each meal should have about 400 calories per day.

Type- meals should be nutritious and protein-rich as well as low in calories and carbs and high in fiber.

Developing own dr now diet plan

The best diet for us is what we develop for ourselves. We have created steps to create your own dr now diet plan. First, make a list of your favorite foods for breakfast, lunch, and dinner. Second, remove all high-calorie foods from the list.

High-calorie foods to avoid:

Sugar, Chocolate, Crackers, Potato chips, Potatoes, French fries, Mashed Potatoes, and tater tots, Popcorn, Peanut butter, almonds, cashews, Pistachios, Sunflower seeds

Candy, cookies, cake, donuts, pies, ice cream, sweetened fruit, and frozen yogurt. Sherbet/sorbet, milkshakes, chocolate milk, pudding, and sweetened gelatin desserts
 White rice and brown rice, Pasta and noodles, cereals

Fruit juices like orange juice, apple juice, cranberry juice, and grape juice.

Bread and tortillas, sodas or sugary drinks or energy drinks

Fruits like watermelon, cantaloupes, and bananas.

Honey syrup, molasses, and meal supplements have excessive carbohydrates and sugar in them.

The third step is to choose, mix and match our favorite food with 400 calories per meal.

4 ounces of grilled chicken breast has 187 calories.
4 ounces of tuna have 209 calories.
One cup of tomato soup has 72 calories.
One boiled egg has 78 calories.
One cup of fat-free yogurt has 95 calories.
So, with very little effort and some homework, we can create our favorite diet plan that is nutritional, satisfying, and sustainable. So far, our own diet is the best diet.

How To Use This Book (Like you've not used any other diet book)

Doctor Nowzaradan Diet is a scientifically proven diet plan. Don't treat this diet plan as just another fad diet. In this book, we focus on your sustainable weight loss. This book gives practical advice on the difficulties faced in losing weight. This book tries to change your bad eating habits into healthy eating habits. The aim is to reduce your weight to a healthy weight and lead a healthy life.

The Sixteen Myths They Want Us To Believe

Myth 1: Restricting Calories For Losing Weight Always Works

One thing most diet plans have in common is calorie restriction. There is almost universal dietary advice "Eat less than required to create a calorie deficit in the body, This will reduce your body fat". But eating fewer calories is based on guesswork. We have no accurate way of knowing how many calories we are eating and burning.

A person who has more muscle mass will burn more calories during any activity. If you eat more protein, your metabolic rate increases. So if you eat fewer calories and get more protein, you burn more calories than someone who eats more calories but less protein.

Myth 2: The Pyramid Of Food Lies

Making the wrong food choice can make you overweight and sick or worse. Making the right food choice is a daily health decision you make. The federal government and every expert will tell you to follow the principles of the food pyramid, but there is not a single study that shows that following the principles of the food pyramid leads to a healthier body weight or better overall health.

Diet varies from region to region and season to season so there is no one formula that we all should follow. What you should not eat is more important than what you should eat. Some early ancestral diets were heavy on plants while others consisted primarily of animal products, yet both ancestors thrived despite having different diets.

A few hundred years ago, none of our ancestors ate anything other than grains, low-fat dairy, and high levels of sugar and processed starches. Your DNA is not yet capable of using these products to keep your body healthy and lean. Obesity rates have risen steadily since the introduction of the USDA Food Pyramid. I searched the internet and couldn't find any research that proves the food pyramid does anything positive for your health.

The USDA Food Pyramid guidelines tell many medical lies. This pyramid of disease encourages you to eat less mass, less vegetables, less fat, more starch, and more dairy food. However, the government is inclined to do so, allowing the USDA to take a look at the suggested food pyramid guidelines before Big Food and Big Agriculture publishes them. Ultimately, the government allowed for-profit corporations to make changes that made the guidelines more acceptable from the perspective of the corporation, its board of directors, and its future profitability.

When the proposed food pyramid came back from the corporation, it was violated to protect their profits. Subsequent guidelines recommended six to eleven servings of grains per day (up from five) and only two to three servings of fruit (up from five to nine). Dairy had earned a section of its own, as if it were an essential food category for all humans, even though 80 percent of people on the planet were unable to consume dairy products. Also, processed and "junk" foods were lumped in with natural, whole foods in all guide sections.

Myth 3: Does Drinking Water Make You Lose Weight?

Drinking water is part of a balanced diet and can help you lose weight, but drinking water alone will not help you lose weight. If you're hungry, it's probably water-induced thirst. Water does not contain any sugar or calories, making it a healthier alternative to sugary or caffeinated drinks.

If you replace your daily intake of beverages like milk, soft drinks, juice etc with water, you will reduce your daily calorie intake as water contains zero calories. For some people, drinking water is a great way to suppress hunger. Water has no weight loss properties. Water takes up space in your stomach and makes you feel full.

It doesn't matter whether your daily water intake is cold or lukewarm, and you don't always need to drink eight glasses of water a day. Drinking water alone will not make you lose weight but drinking enough water will keep you healthy and hydrated, boosts energy and aids digestion and prevents bloating. Water is essential for good health.

Myth 4: Fiber Is Necessary For A Healthy Gut

Everyone, your parents, doctors and nutritionists keep telling you fiber is good for you. The Big food industry also loves this lie because it's easy for them to add a little fiber to the junk food they're selling and then label the boxes with high fiber levels. People tell you that consuming more fiber can prevent constipation, diverticulosis and colon cancer.

There are several observational studies that support this hypothesis. Although observational studies have shown a correlation between increased fiber intake and constipation, diverticulosis and decreased rates of colon cancer, observational studies do not prove causation. Also, observational studies have measured dietary fiber from vegetables and fruits rather than added fiber from other industrial junk foods. Fiber is plant material that passes through the digestive tract and is excreted in the stool.

Virtually all research that says eating more fiber is good for you is in the form of observational studies that don't prove causation. This is not enough evidence for doctors and dieticians to tell patients to eat more fiber. One review article found that the less fiber participants ate, the less constipation they experienced. Participants who ate the most fiber had more severe symptoms of constipation than those in the study who ate no fiber at all. Two large studies show no benefits for colon health from eating more dietary fiber.

I never go out of my way to eat more fiber. In fact there are plenty of days each week when I don't notice any fiber at all. I do occasionally eat some vegetables but rarely do I eat more than a few grams of fiber. Even if I eat very little fiber.

Myth 5: Fad Diets Works If You Follow Them

Is this a lie? People stop following diets because their rules are too difficult. Many diet plans require you to do things that are not sustainable. Like I was in my twenties you will lose weight quickly but that is their business model they know you will come back because once you get off the impossible diet restrictions you will gain the weight back if you were born addicted to sugar and processed food.

It will take more than a month of crash dieting to reverse the conditioning that makes you sick. Also, I don't give you a fad diet to follow in this book, I teach you sustainable lifestyle changes that you can stick with for life and that keep your weight under control and lead a healthy life. If you succeed in my program you won't need me. I don't want repeat customers like everyone else.

I see other people who have been taking medicine continuously for five, ten, fifteen years and follow one fad diet one after another. Medicines are a subscription product. Big Pharma is not in the business of selling you products you won't need anytime soon. Sustainable diet changes don't make you sad. You can eat in a way that makes you feel full without feeling hungry and still be healthy. The truth is that there is no ideal human diet. One diet cannot suit every person.

Myth 6: Weight Loss Diets Work For Long-Term Weight Loss

95 percent of diet plans are not successful, but why you should try to lose weight. Every one of our fellow neighbors have friends and family who have lost weight but it is impossible for them to lose weight continuously. Some people have a sluggish thyroid or a naturally slow metabolism. Another reason is that some people's metabolism slows down, forcing your body to gain weight even if you eat less.

There's a lot of food around us that's high in calories and tastes good, and it's heavily advertised. Both low activity and palatable food can make sustained weight loss a challenge. Sustained weight loss requires four things: choosing the right diet, being physically active, making positive lifestyle changes, and Creating a supportive environment. It is important to choose the right diet. People who follow certain strategies while choosing food are on the path to permanent weight loss.

Keep these things in mind when making food choices:
1. Keep the foods you want to eat always available
2. Use fresh fruits and vegetables
3. Start the day on a healthy note
4. Plan healthy snacks
5. Make the right choices for dozens of other simple recipes

Focus on daily exercise. Choose an exercise you like and do it regularly. Create a Supportive Environment. A supportive environment is essential for losing weight and keeping it off. Telling the people who care about you that you're losing weight can help you. There are many people who achieve sustainable weight loss because they choose the right diet, are physically active, live a healthy lifestyle with a positive mindset, and are in a supportive environment.

Myth 7: Should I Focus Mostly On Exercise?

According to the researchers, over-eating and less exercise are responsible for the weight gain over the past thirty years. Our body needs movement because our body is not designed to sit still in one place. Lack of exercise leads to weight gain. Weight gain occurs when more calories are consumed than expended in activity. Beyond its role in weight control, exercise improves overall health.

If you take in more calories than you burn, you gain weight, and when you burn more calories than you take in, you lose weight. To lose 1 pound of weight you need to create a deficit of 3500 calories. A deficit of 500 calories per day should be created in a week. You can make up for this deficiency by eating less food and exercising more, but how much exercise should be involved?

People who start an exercise program often neglect the food side of the equation calorie in= calorie out. It also increases the amount of food they eat as they feel they are burning more calories than they are taking in. The end result is weight gain instead of weight loss.

Losing two pounds per week without changing your diet requires continuing to do everything you are currently doing plus walking an extra 10 mile per day which means a lot of exercise and time. Several panels of experts looked at all the evidence and came to the conclusion that although exercise is extremely important, exercise alone does not lead to significant weight loss. It is possible that the weight can stay the same during a weight loss program because exercise builds muscle and muscle weighs more than fat.

Myth 8: What Counts The Most—Fats, Carbs, Or Calories?

A balanced diet that provides the right amount of nutritious carbohydrates and fats can help with weight loss and long-term weight maintenance. Such a diet includes all food groups. A balanced diet contains the right amount of fat for heart health along with the recommended fiber levels.

Both fats and carbohydrates are nutrients that our body needs. In addition, these macronutrients provide additional nutrients such as vitamins, minerals and phytochemicals and reduce the risk of many diseases. There are a lot of food choices available for fat and carbs, the key is choosing the right food without following a diet. Researchers suggest that those who have lost weight can successfully maintain a balanced diet that includes the recommended levels of fat and carbohydrates.

Food weight and health are interrelated topics. A balanced diet is a good way to balance these three. When you deplete macronutrients, you remove essential nutrients and potential health benefits they can provide. From here on, choose foods that contain healthy fats such as polyunsaturated, monounsaturated and omega-3 fatty acids. Reduce your intake of trans fats by limiting baked goods, cookies, crackers, and fried foods. Reduce saturated fats by choosing low-fat dairy products. Nutritious sources of carbohydrates include low-fat dairy products, legumes, whole grains and grain products, fresh fruit. Create the food balance that works best for you.

Myth 9: All Calories Are Created Equal

It's a misconception that all calories are the same. For example, the amount of calories in between birthday cake and broccoli varies.

It is patently false that if you burn the same number of calories as you consume each day, you will maintain the same weight. Because it is not only useful to count calories to lose weight but also what kind of food we are eating is important. It is important to know how many calories your body eats each day and get them from nutritious food. Because both the amount of calories and nutrients in food are important to our body.

To maintain good health we must know what is really important to us. If you want a strong mind and a healthy body, what should you spend your money and effort on? Many doctors tell their patients that in order to lose weight, we must burn more calories than we consume. But doctors are unknowingly lying because not all calories are created equal. Some foods are high in calories and some foods are unable to provide nutrition to the body. Therefore, eating such foods does not benefit the body.

Doctors are very busy and most of them don't realize that learning about nutrition is more important to the health of their patients than learning about the newest pill from Big Pharma. A doctor does not aim to be a nutritionist but rather an expert in drugs and medical procedures. Don't worry about the amount of calories you eat. Eating the wrong foods and disrupting your insulin metabolism can lead to weight gain. - Not because of eating too many calories.

Myth 10: Starve Yourself To Lose Weight

Crash dieting does not result in long term weight loss but often results in long-term weight gain. The real problem is that it's very difficult to follow this kind of diet. Following a crash diet will leave your body low on energy and cause you to crave more high-fat and high-sugar foods, which can lead to weight gain as you overeat and consume more calories than you need.

It's a common misconception that starving yourself and skipping meals accelerates your weight loss journey. No matter what the fad diet claims, starving yourself and skipping meals is not a sustainable weight loss strategy. Instead always eat at regular intervals so you stay fuller for longer and keep a safe distance from fried and fatty foods.

Myth 11: Eating At Night Makes You Gain Weight Calories

Your weight does not depend on the time you eat. If you don't eat more calories than your body needs and eat dinner late, you won't gain weight. But eating dinner early also has many benefits. Eating dinner early helps your body settle down, which can prevent indigestion before bed. It can also help you sleep better.

A lot also depends on what we eat. Eating late at night and choosing high calorie and unhealthy foods at night can lead to weight gain. But if you eat healthy and nutritious food in the evening, you can lead a healthy life.

Myth 12: Skipping Breakfast Helps You Lose Weight

Skipping or eating breakfast does not help in weight loss. According to the researchers, there was no correlation between breakfast habits and weight loss. Also, eating breakfast in the morning can make you feel fuller for longer. The saying that breakfast is the most important meal may or may not be true. But skipping breakfast does not necessarily help in weight loss. Skipping breakfast does not necessarily reduce total caloric intake for the day.

Myth 13: Going Gluten-Free Is The Solution To Weight Loss

Gluten free foods are low in fiber. So you don't feel full for a long time. The amount of food you eat can increase. Many processed foods are higher in fat and sugar than gluten-free ingredients. Eating such food can also make you gain weight.

Gluten is a type of protein found in certain grains. Like wheat, barley and rye. People with celiac are at risk of gluten. Gluten itself is not dangerous for the rest of us and is found in many healthy foods that are also high in fiber, vitamins and minerals.

Myth 14: Juice Cleanses Work

Juice cleans are considered a way to lose weight. When your body is running low on calories and you're depriving yourself and that's never a good idea. Eating too much liquid sugar can cause your blood sugar to rise and cause you to gain weight. Even if you lose weight, after a few days your body goes into conservation mode and regaining the weight you lost is just another thing that your body is doing on a juice cleanse.

While on a juice cleanse remember that juices are generally high in calories so it's best to keep your intake in moderation. There are also health risks such as kidney problems, possible dehydration due to empty intestines, electrolyte imbalances, etc

Everyone thinks that a juice cleanse is a quick way to lose weight, but it's not. Even though you're consuming fewer calories, you're also consuming a lot of sugar, which can spike your blood sugar and cause weight gain.

Myth 15: Do My Genes Or Metabolism Keep Me From Achieving Sustainable Weight Loss?

Weight loss and sustained weight loss are not the same for everyone. We are all different We are simply born with our own genetic makeup. We make life choices and develop a personal biology that affects our ability to lose weight long-term. Some people are born with fat genes, their mom and dad are fat, their grandparents are fat, and their cousins are fat. People who come from large families have no choice but to being big too. Then there is a life event that causes weight gain that cannot be reversed.

Metabolism affects the rate of weight loss and people have different metabolic rates. One way to lose weight is to increase the metabolism by improving the body's engine so that it burns more calories. Any way of getting ready to move will burn off more calories. Some experts say that an overweight parent has at least a 40% chance of being overweight.

Obesity researchers believe there is a strong link between a person's genetic makeup and their vulnerability to weight gain. But the human genome, or genetic map, changes very slowly—perhaps less than one percent every million years—how can we explain why obesity rates in the United States have increased by 40 percent in the past decade?

For those who seek the right balance between food and exercise to lose weight, having fat genes doesn't matter. Biology is not luck. Many different factors influence weight loss, but no single factor prevents weight loss. It is true that some people have a genetic or personal profile that makes them more vulnerable to weight gain, yet prevent weight gain and gain more weight. Sustained weight loss is possible for virtually anyone.

Myth 16: Is Weight A Good Indicator Of Health?

Weight is relative. A six-foot-tall man and a five-foot-tall woman may each weigh two hundred pounds, but they look and feel very different when carrying it. This suggests that there is some correlation between weight and height. So to look more objectively at weight and health, health experts calculate weight in relation to height called body mass index or BMI.

The trouble with BMI is that it doesn't take into account how the weight was formed. Even people with not a lot of muscle can fall into the overweight or obese category. For example, even if they have less body fat. People with very little muscle mass may have a normal weight-for-height ratio but have high blood pressure, high cholesterol, and chronic disease.

Some researchers have found that being slightly overweight can be healthier than being slightly underweight. The short answer to whether weight is a good indicator of health is no because it must be combined with other factors to get a true sense of your health. Body fat percentage is a useful health indicator measured by special scales or equipment in clinics and doctor's offices. The more fat tissue you have, the more fat your body needs. The more fat tissue you have, the harder it is for your body to do basic functions like converting glucose into fuel and pumping blood through your veins.

Excess weight is often a side effect of unhealthy habits and a warning sign of potential complications, but a few pounds won't doom you to a life of chronic disease. How you feel, how you eat, and how you move are always more important than the number on the scale.

Why Do People Fail at Weight Loss?

This is a good question because some fail. People who go on diet plans say that we find it difficult to break our old habits and adopt new healthy habits. We can understand because initially when we leave our comfort zone, we feel a little uncomfortable. But if we are determined and if we keep following our diet plan, we can definitely succeed.

When we are in the first 30 days of our diet plan, we lose 9 to 14 pounds. When we try to make healthy habits, we have a lot of chances of failure because it requires self control and mental preparation to give up high calorie and tasty food, and exercise daily.

People who lose weight after 30 days feel like their weight loss is permanent and now they can add some tasty food to their diet plan and it won't make much of a difference. But they don't even realize that a little bit of tasty food sometimes turns into a lot of tasty food. So these people don't even realize that they are consuming more calories than the daily requirement.

Emotional Eating- Emotional eating is a condition where a person eats to feel good and to relieve stress rather than to satisfy hunger. In emotional eating, people choose foods that are high in fat, sugar, trans fat, and other toxic ingredients. It is a fact that 95% diet plan and 5% exercise are important in weight loss but we are wrong to give more importance to exercise. Ignoring or misreading label information can increase your calorie intake and hinder weight loss.

Part 2

Shift Mindset From Diet To Lifestyle

When we decide to improve our health, we must follow a system. We should follow some principles from here on in life so that we can control the weight and lead a healthy life. These principles are derived from my own experience and from the results of research on people. As I followed these principles, I began to see them working. Let us now discuss each principle.

Principle 1 - Let's create a system for our health and let go of trying to reach any kind of goal.

The first step to creating a diet plan is to get out of the diet and weight loss mindset. When most people decide to live a healthy life, they set a goal without thinking it through. For example, if a person is fat and has fat around his waist, he decides that I want to lose so many inches from my waist. But we have observed that even thin individuals can have a poor metabolism as a result of which they cannot live a healthy life.

So we should not set short term goals for our body. We should adopt healthy habits with a lifelong mindset. The first is because the goal mindset doesn't work. For example, let's say you decide to lose 20 pounds, and after following some restrictions, you lose that much weight, but you feel that you are now free to eat your favorite, high-calorie foods, resulting in the weight you lost gaining back.

We need to change our mindset to stay healthy. It is very important to know the purpose of why we want to live a healthy life. I think my aim should be that I will live a long and good life with my system. Also in my opinion it is the best system that you can follow again and again without thinking. Rather than chasing multiple goals at once, we need to stick to one system. I have dealt with this goal mentality myself. I did the math on what a healthy weight is for me and decided that I needed to lose 35 pounds to reach a healthy weight. I tried to lose weight repeatedly and lost some of it but gained it back.

After this experience I created a system to live a healthy life and decided to focus on maintaining health. I stopped the habit of losing weight every day and started focusing on how my health was changing. Once you learn to follow systems instead of goals, dealing with medical and metabolic health becomes much less intimidating.

8

Principle 2: Get into the habit of eating whole foods.

Are you wondering what is a whole food? The answer is not as difficult as you think. Most of the food we eat has a label that states what ingredients are in the food. Note that food is an element in itself. Whole foods are foods that we can grow in our backyards, as well as think about what foods our grandparents would have been eating a hundred years ago. The food they ate in their time was called whole food. In short, unprocessed food is whole food.

There are certain nutritional needs of our body that we must fulfill. Your body should be stimulated to survive. That's what tells your brain when your stomach is full. I am not a fan of labels. My goal is not to make you stick to a diet. So the switch from fake processed food to real food is. Remember we are building a system. Not focusing on any goal. I never say that I never eat that food. I usually avoid it. This method has an advantage. Everyone likes to eat ice cream. For example, when we follow a diet, we eat the foods it says and avoid foods like ice cream.

We give up after trying so hard and then we feel like a failure. I eat ice cream but I eat ice cream made with simple ingredients. And try to reduce the effect of ice cream by fasting the next day. I am not telling you to live life without things like ice cream, we have to set priorities in our life. Healthy food should be given first place in our diet so that we can live a healthy life.

Principle 3: Make one sustainable change at a time.

You must know the pareto principle which states that for many results 80% of the results come from 20% of the causes. It means that the results of the system that we are going to build to live a healthy life are only 20% of the causes. So if we are going to make one change at a time, it will be beneficial for us to find the best change. We are going to tell you some important changes that will benefit you the best. Prioritize. Get into the habit of eating real whole foods first. Most people gravitate towards carbohydrates and foods high in sugar. Because they like the taste of those foods. There is a solution to do so. Make it a habit to eat whole foods instead of the sugary foods and carbs you eat. This requires a change in your mindset and a bit of work. Instead of spending the last 10 to 20 years of your life stuck in an electric wheelchair, what's wrong with getting your body used to working a little harder now?

Instead of cooking with fake oils, use highly processed and industrial oils like safflower oil, canola oil, sunflower oil - real whole foods. The last suggestion is to eat less snacks. Real whole foods that are nutritionally dense at mealtimes make you feel full for a long time. On the other hand, if we eat packaged food, we feel hungry again within 1 hour. If your body doesn't get what it needs, it sends you hunger signals to snack to get the rest of your body's nutrients. When we include nutrient-dense foods in our meals, we feel full and don't need to snack as often. It helps in weight loss. Start by making these changes one at a time.

Principle 4: Exercise

Now is the time to be active throughout the day. Due to modern lifestyle, we spend more time sitting during the day. Why do we eat food or take in calories? Because we should use those calories but we are used to sitting all day long. And when we get bored of sitting we eat breakfast. This breakfast adds calories to the body without burning any calories. Instead of exercising for 1-2 hours once a day, make it a habit to exercise in small intervals throughout the day to get more movement. Be more active whenever possible. I'm going to tell you some ways you can be more active.

1. Take the stairs instead of the elevator.
2. Park the car far away and make it a habit to walk more.
3. Make it a habit to play actively with your children and pets.
4. Go for a morning or evening walk with a partner.
5. Make it a habit to listen to an audiobook while walking to read a book.

You will burn more calories if you are active throughout the day than if you are sedentary all day, working out in the gym for an hour, sleeping for eight hours, and sitting for fifteen hours. Building and maintaining muscle as you age should be the primary focus. Because it is directly related to the quality of life. Research shows that cardio is an incredible fat loss tactic.

Principle 5: Get enough sleep

Did you read properly? Get enough sleep. You must have thought that getting enough sleep means sleeping longer. Perhaps this is true in a sense but the quality of your sleep is just as important as how long you sleep. You need deep sleep to rest and recover. According to researchers, people who eat nutritious food have better sleep and sleep more deeply. Because it does not destroy your body with bad food. And they lose weight. They cause less stress to the body so they can take less sleep to recover. It also means that you don't feel tired throughout the day. And you don't have to drink coffee in the afternoon to beat the slack. If you feel tired every day, this is not normal.

This could be because you choose carbs and sugary foods instead of nutritious food for your daily meals. Also you will not be able to be active all day. To get good sleep, your sleeping environment needs to be good. Sleep environment depends on how you prepare yourself for sleep. Most people have a habit of looking at their mobile while lying in bed. This is poor sleep hygiene. Because the blue light on your mobile phone is harmful to your brain. That blue light doesn't make you fall asleep quickly. It is not a good habit to look at your mobile for 1 hour before going to bed. You should read paperback books of your choice before going to sleep. Avoid stimulants before bed. Avoid cigarettes and alcohol after meals.

Principle 6: Reduce stress in your life.

Stress causes inflammation and hormonal changes that counteract healthy health. If the stress in your current life is off the charts, you need to take drastic steps to reduce stress. Daily meditation can be a good solution to reduce your stress. For most of us, part of the problem is that we don't add helpful stress-reducing elements to our day. Whichever path you take, mindfulness is a useful practice for grounding yourself in the present rather than worrying about the future. Being intentional about what you're doing throughout the day and reacting thoughtfully rather than reacting immediately can help reduce stress. In short, less stress makes it easier to stay healthy.

What Exactly Is Belly Fat, and Where Does It Come From?

Weight gain can be caused by many reasons, and excess fat on your body can affect your health. The fat that accumulates around your organs, including your stomach, intestines, and liver, is what we call visceral fat. You can't see visceral fat but it's there. Subcutaneous fat that you can see and feel by hand is subcutaneous fat. Subcutaneous fat provides insulation, which serves as storage and has a protective effect between our skin and our muscles and bones.

Most of us know very little about our belly fat. For example, if you look at your childhood photos, you will see fat spread all over your body. Like chubby cheeks, chubby thighs, chubby wrists. As we grow older, these tend to gather around the midsection of the body. Always remember that belly fat is active in spoiling your health.

The fat cells in your belly release hormones and other irritating chemicals into your body. Proteins in them called cytokines contribute to inflammation-related problems. According to Harvard researchers, visceral fat cells secrete high levels of a molecule called RBP4, which increases insulin resistance, which increases the risk of weight gain and diabetes. Therefore, belly fat increases further. This means that the more visceral fat you have, the harder it will be to keep the weight off in the future.

Inflammation is a response to cell damage. Fat cells are swollen and consequently very fragile. They burst and die easily. When they die, they trigger an inflammatory response called inflammation. Inflammation reduces muscle mass. Muscle is very good at storing excess, but if the body loses muscle, the excess calories are stored in belly fat. It increases its thickness. This creates an equation such that more belly fat leads to more inflammation in our body leading to less muscle mass. Loss of muscle mass causes excess calories to be stored in belly fat leading to increased belly fat. This creates a cycle in which our belly fat continues to increase.

Take vitamin B12. Vitamin B 12, found only in animal foods, is essential for building healthy red blood cells. A poor diet and the use of other drugs can damage the ecosystem in our heart. Also, too many artificial chemicals and too much sugar can disrupt the balance of bacteria in our gut. The bacteria that thrive in this disturbed environment increase inflammation in our body. This makes it difficult for us to absorb nutrients, vitamins and minerals from food. An altered microbiome in the body causes us to absorb more calories than a healthy person. Keeping your gut healthy and maintaining a balance of bad bacteria is very important.

How should we take care of our belly?

You should eat fiber to control your belly fat. Fiber is edible but indigestible part of plants. If we eat more fiber, we reduce the risk of 6 major diseases. Such as stroke, heart disease, cancer, respiratory disease, Alzheimer's, and diabetes. Fiber helps prevent bowel obstructions and in doing so reduces the risk of disease, helping your body retain muscle. It also promotes weight loss. But Americans consume only half as much fiber each day.

Good Carb Bad Carb

We always blame carbs for weight gain. But are they true? Some carbs are actually bad but some carbs are actually good. Good carbohydrates provide fuel for your body. Carbs that occur naturally in plant-based foods are good carbs. These types of carbs promote a healthy metabolism and digestive system. Bad carbs are found in processed foods. These are called simple carbs that are absorbed into the bloodstream and become blood sugar.

There are two types of carbohydrates. Simple and complex carbohydrates Simple carbohydrates are harmful to the body. Simple carbohydrates are digested quickly and raise blood sugar levels. Which makes us hungry quickly. Due to this, we develop diseases like weight gain, high blood pressure, diabetes.

Complex carbohydrates are the good kind. They are full of fiber. This slows down the digestion process in your body and prevents blood sugar levels. If you choose whole grains instead of white rice, white bread, and pastries for your carbs right now, you get two benefits, one is the benefits of complex carbs and you're less likely to eat processed foods that spike blood sugar.

Carbohydrates fall into 3 more groups. Fiber, starch and sugar
Fiber comes from plant-based foods. Fiber helps your intestines digest other nutrients. It makes you feel full for longer. Helps you lose weight by avoiding overeating.

quinoa and oats, nuts and seeds, beans and lentils, brown rice and pasta

Starches are also a type of complex carbohydrates. Like fiber, they are also digested slowly. And they provide essential vitamins and minerals to the body.
Vegetables, legumes, beans, fruits
There are two types of sugar, natural and added
Our body does not know the difference between natural and added sugar. Our mind doesn't know the difference between the sugar in fruit and the sugar in a donut, but fruit also gives us other nutrients that donuts don't.

Looking at all this, the benefits of healthy carbohydrates become clear to us. Not consuming healthy carbohydrates can affect your body. Carbohydrates provide fuel for many organs in the body. By fueling the brain, central nervous system, digestive system, these organs become stronger, it helps prevent diseases like heart disease and diabetes.

Also, such carbohydrates are stored in the body. It gives the body fuel when you don't consume carbohydrates. Not consuming enough carbohydrates can cause diseases in our body. Giving up bad carbs can be difficult but not impossible. You can change your habits by making small changes. Like using whole grain bread instead of white bread. Choose 'whole' carbohydrates to stay healthy and as close to their natural state as possible.

Good Fat Bad Fat

When we think of diet, we think of fat as an ingredient for our body, but not all fats play a role in obesity, cancer, diabetes. Not all fats are good for your body. Some fats are better than others. They help promote good health. Knowing the difference between good fats and bad fats can help us plan which fats to avoid and which ones to consume less. Saturated fat and trans fat are two types of fat considered potentially harmful to your body. Most of these substances are solid at room temperature.

butter

Beef or pork

We should avoid trans fat and eat very little saturated fat.

Saturated fat includes beef, pork, chicken, meat and poultry, as well as high-fat dairy products.

Eating too much saturated fat can increase blood cholesterol levels. According to researchers, if people replace saturated fat with polyunsaturated fat, your risk of heart disease may decrease.

Avoid trans fat whenever possible. These include fried foods (french fries, fried fast food), baked foods (cookies, pastries), processed snacks.

According to doctors, trans fats can have harmful effects on our body, including heart disease, diabetes and stroke.

Bad trans fat

Trans fats have no health benefits and should not be consumed in moderation. So it has been officially banned in America. Eating foods high in trans fats increases the amount of cholesterol in the bloodstream. Trans fats increase the risk of diabetes, heart disease, stroke. Consuming even a small amount of trans fat can cause harm to the body.

Nutrition Info

One pound of fat provides your body with 3500 calories. Most women burn 1800 to 2100 calories. Most men burn between 2100 and 2600 calories. To lose 1 pound of fat per week, the average woman would need to cut calorie intake by 1/4 and men by 1/5. Reducing body fat should be considered a long-term process, not a short-term one. But our body needs constant energy. The food you eat gives your body energy. A balance needs to be maintained between the energy we get from food and the energy we burn through activity. This is the basic principle of weight control.

The energy we take into the body through food is measured in units called calories. Finding calories in a food list is easy. Energy burned during activity is also measured in units called calories. Lists are also available for that. Tracking calories in and calories out in a journal is helpful for weight loss. The food you eat contains a variety of macronutrients that provide the energy your body needs.

These macronutrients include carbohydrates, fats, and proteins. Other nutrients required by the body like vitamins, minerals do not provide calories but help in chemical processes. Carbohydrates can be simple or complex. Simple carbohydrates are found in fruits, honey, milk, dairy products and complex carbohydrates are found in whole grains, potatoes, pasta, beans and vegetables. Complex carbohydrates contain many vitamins and minerals, fiber.

Complex carbohydrates are stripped of many of their nutrients and benefits during processing. There are different types of fats. Cooking oil is a type of fat. Fat is a major source of calories. Proteins build and repair body structures. Excess protein also provides calories. Proteins are made up of basic building blocks called amino acids.

Fresh organic food is rich in nutrients. Minerals like calcium, magnesium and phosphorus are important for teeth and bones. Electrolytes, such as sodium, potassium, and chloride, help regulate chemical balance and water in our bodies. Minerals like iodine, zinc, iron, fluoride, manganese and selenium that our body needs in small amounts are called trace minerals.

Water is an important element for our body. Many foods, especially fruits, contain a lot of water. Drinking water has many benefits. Like drinking water keeps body temperature under control. Helps carry nutrients and oxygen in the bloodstream. It also helps in carrying waste.

Fiber- Fiber is part of plant foods, our body cannot absorb fiber. There are two types of fiber soluble and insoluble. Soluble foods include apples, citrus fruits, dried peas, beans, barley, and oatmeal. Soluble fiber lowers cholesterol which reduces blood sugar spikes. Insoluble fiber is found in whole grains, wheat bran, bread, pasta, cereals, and many vegetables.

What is a calorie?
A calorie is a unit used to measure any energy. We use calories to measure nutrition. Food energy is measured in kilocalories.

Carbohydrates are the first nutrients your body uses. As our body digests them, they are released into the bloodstream and converted into glucose, or blood sugar. When your body needs energy, glucose is immediately absorbed into your body's cells to provide energy. Glucose can be stored in your liver and muscles if there is no current demand. When these storage sites are full, excess glucose is converted to fatty acids and stored in fat tissue for later use. Fat is the best form of energy and packs the most calories.

After digestion they break down into fatty acids. Excess fatty acids can also be stored in your muscles. There is no limit to how much fat can be stored in our body. Protein also contains calories. Vitamins, water, minerals and fiber have no calories. However, they are important for our health. When they are lacking in our diet, we are more prone to serious illnesses.

Food sources of energy
Fat alone provides more calories than protein and carbohydrates together.

You can understand your energy needs and costs from the example of your bank account. Suppose you have a bank account and you transact through it every day. Your deposit is food that contains three types of nutrients: carbohydrates, proteins, and fats. When you eat food, you add calories to your body. You can withdraw money from your account in three ways. One of them is BMR Basal Metabolic Rate – the amount of calories your body burns even when you are at rest. As your body uses energy to meet basic needs such as respiration, circulation, cellular growth and repair. This is called BMR i.e. Basal Metabolic Rate. BMR is responsible for the most caloric expenditure.

The energy used to digest, absorb, transport and store the food you eat is known as the thermic effect of food and is another form of calorie burning. Physical Activity – The activities we do with our bodies every day also require energy. Our body's BMR and digestive needs remain relatively constant and are not easy to change. One of the best ways to burn your calories is to increase your physical activity.

If every human being were physically and functionally identical, it would be easy to determine the amount of energy required for each person's activities. But other factors affect your energy bill. Age, body size, composition, and gender are some of the factors that affect energy requirements and BMR.

Childrens are in the process of developing muscles, bones, and need more calories per pound. Just as body composition changes with age, so does your BMR. As you reach middle age, your energy needs decrease. Muscle burns more calories than fat, so the more muscle you have in your body, the higher your BMR.

Men have less body fat and more muscle than women of the same age and weight. Therefore men have higher BMR and energy requirements than women.

Balancing your account.

How well your body's energy balance is known by looking at your weight. Daily changes in your weight reflect changes in your energy balance. If you burn the same number of calories as you take in through food every day, your weight will stay the same. If you expend more calories than you burn, you lose weight, and if you expend fewer calories than you burn, you gain weight. A magic number in calorie expenditure and accumulation is 3500 calories because 3500 calories equals 1 pound of fat. If you want to burn 1 pound of fat, you need to burn 3500 calories more. As the amount of food we eat on a daily basis changes, so does the amount of calories in our body. Therefore, there is no balance between the calories coming and expending in our body.

You should keep track of how many calories you consume from what you eat, drink, and how many calories you burn through physical activity. It can help you lose weight. But we can't follow this for a long time rather we should focus on weight control. To lose weight, you can build your body by eating fewer calories, burning more calories through physical activity, or both. The best way to do this is to eat healthy and be active. We should adopt a healthy lifestyle.

What is the science behind it?

What the first law of thermodynamics tells us is that energy is neither created nor destroyed, energy is simply transferred from one form to another. The calories you eat are either converted into physical energy or stored in the body. All unused calories in your body become fat, regardless of where they come from. The energy balance equation is easy to understand in theory but difficult to follow. We gain or lose weight only because of energy imbalance.
But weight control can become easier if we understand the concept of energy balance. If you can eat foods that provide plenty of weight and volume but not a lot of calories, you can feel fuller while losing or maintaining weight. So when we follow a 1200 calorie diet, we should eat more protein to make us feel fuller for longer on fewer calories.

Fast food, soda, candies, simple sugar, processed foods are high in energy density. Other foods do not contain many calories. Energy density is low among vegetables and fruits. Let's take an example: a candy bar contains 280 calories, while most raw vegetables contain 25 calories. If you eat foods that are low in energy density, it can help you lose weight.

Research suggests that whether your stomach is full is determined by the amount and weight of food. Not on the number of calories you eat. According to the researchers, people who ate a low energy density diet were able to lose weight. By choosing foods that are low in energy density, you can consume fewer calories and lose weight even when you are full.

Vegetables
Vegetables include greens, spinach, carrots, beets, radishes, cabbage, and 25 calories in one bowl. Vegetables are low in cholesterol and low in fat and sodium. Vegetables are high in magnesium and potassium.

Fruits
One fruit contains about 60 calories and fruits are virtually fat free. Like vegetables, fruits are a great source of fiber, vitamins, minerals and other phytochemicals. So fruits can help you lose weight and reduce the risk of weight related diseases.

carbohydrates
Most carbohydrates are plant-based. They include starchy foods like potatoes, corn, and cereals, bread, and pasta. But what carbohydrates should we focus on and eat? It is very easy to determine. Choose foods that are less processed, such as whole grain breads, pastas and cereals. The key word in carbohydrates is whole, generally speaking the less refined the carbohydrate food, the better it is for you.

protein
Your bones, muscles, skin, and organ tissues are made of protein. Proteins are often associated with food of animal origin, but they are also found in plants. Protein is found in foods such as legumes, fish, chicken, and lean meat. Whole milk dairy products are good sources of protein and calcium. Beans, lentils and peas are excellent sources of protein. Research suggests that most people will benefit from eating at least two servings of fish per week.

fats
You may not believe it but fats are essential for the life and function of your body's cells. In addition to storing energy, fats play an important role in the immune system and help maintain cell structure. Examples of good fat sources are cooking oil, avocados, seeds, olives, and nuts. Fats are high in calories. So we should take less.

Finding Your Healthy Weight

You know you need to lose weight and you have a reason to lose it. That reason may be to look good but keep this reason aside and focus on another important factor. Think about your health. Having a good weight for your health can also be called a healthy weight. You can reduce the risk of various skin diseases in the future. Your life can be extended and your emotions can improve.

What is a healthy weight?

A healthy weight is the right amount of body fat you have in relation to total body mass. This weight makes us feel energetic, reduces health risks, helps prevent premature aging and improves quality of life. Stepping on the scale tells us our total weight, not our fat percentage. We don't even know where this fat is going. The most accurate way to determine how much fat you are carrying is to do a body fat analysis.

Body mass index is a tool that shows your weight status. Height and weight are taken into account while calculating BMI. Although BMI does not differentiate between fat and muscle, it more accurately reflects body fat than total body weight.

To determine your BMI, find your height in the left column. Follow that row up to your nearest weight. Look at the top of that column for your estimated BMI. Or use this formula.

Formula: weight (lb) / [height (in)]2 x 703

Calculate BMI by dividing weight in pounds (lbs) by height in inches (in) squared and multiplying by a conversion factor of 703.

There is a relationship between excess weight and the location of body fat. Fat distribution is in two types of shapes, apple shape or pear shape. If you carry most of your fat around your waist or upper body, consider yourself apple-shaped. If most of your fat is around your thighs or lower waist, consider yourself pear shaped. In general it is better to be pear shaped than apple shaped. Measure around your waist. Measurements greater than 40 inches in men or 35 inches in women indicate apple size and increased health risks. It is important to know that the larger the waistline, the greater the risks to your health.

How To Eat In A Restaurant

Eating out is sometimes necessary. And by adopting a few healthy habits, you can enjoy eating out without packing on extra pounds. You just need to be menu savvy to eat out. When eating at a restaurant it is important to be aware of the food you are eating as the ingredients are not labeled on the food. The extra calories come from ingredients we don't know about. That is why it is a problem for people who are under weight control. Many ingredients are added to give food flavor and color to food.

People who are trying to change their eating habits are afraid to go out to eat at restaurants. Because here people are encouraged to consume sugar and carbohydrates. Remember you need a sustainable eating plan, not a restrictive one.

Use these tips to eliminate hidden calories and fat in restaurants.

When you go out to a restaurant, make sure to eat real whole foods rather than processed foods. Order 2 or 3 burger patties without a bun instead of a burger and fries. Among the carbs you can order steak. And can have a baked potato with biscuits and green beans. Eat a little at home before going to a restaurant so you don't get too hungry. Alfredo sauce may be full of harmful ingredients and you may not even know it.

You can always just ask and make specific requests while in a restaurant. It is not rude to ask a server in a restaurant for a list of ingredients and to prepare your food in a particular way. Ask for your fish to be prepared in butter rather than in vegetable oil or margarine. Don't be shy about asking for what you want. To stay healthy, we should eat food according to healthy habits. Don't think about eating constantly. Pay attention to the experience of eating in a restaurant, you won't remember what you ate in 10 years. If you can prepare good tasting and healthy food at home, you won't have the same urge to go to a restaurant. Someone else prepares the food but you have to bear the consequences in your body and in your life when you eat it.

Appetizers- If you are going to choose an appetizer, choose one that consists mainly of vegetables, fruits or fish. Avoid fried or breaded appetizers. Soup- Choose tomato based or broth based while choosing soup. Bread– Muffins, garlic toast and croissants contain more calories and fat than whole grain bread, breadsticks and crackers. Request the server to bring a breadbasket to avoid cravings for bread. Salad- Lettuce or spinach salad is good for you. Also beware of addons that are high in calories.

Avoid chef salad and taco salad if possible as they are high in calories. Choose fresh fruits, steamed vegetables, rice, baked or boiled potatoes as a side dish instead of high calorie foods. Dessert- Finish your main dish before ordering dessert. If you order dessert, share it with one of your companions. Optionally order fresh fruit or sherbet for dessert.

Avoid these terms : breaded, broasted, buttered, creamed, fried
Look for these terms: Baked, broiled, Grilled, Poached, Roasted, Sauted, Steamed

Soft drinks or alcoholic beverages add extra calories. So take water in the restaurant if possible.

YOUR GUIDE TO HEALTHY ETHNIC CUISINE

These suggestions will help you savor the exotic, while keeping calories, fat, cholesterol and sodium under control.

Chinese

Look for: Stir-fried or steamed dishes with lots of vegetables, steamed rice, poached fish, and hot and sour soups.

Avoid: Fatty spareribs, fried wontons, egg rolls, shrimp toast and fried rice. To limit sodium, ask that your food be prepared without salt or monosodium glutamate (MSG). Request soy sauce (high in sodium) and other sauces on the side.

French

Look for: Steamed shellfish, roasted poultry, salad with dressing on the side, and sauces with a wine or tomato base, such as bordelaise or à la Provençal.

Avoid: French onion soup (high in sodium; high in fat if it has cheese), high-fat sauces (béchamel, hollandaise and béarnaise), croissants and pâte.

Greek

Look for: Plaki (fish cooked with tomatoes, onions and garlic), chicken kebabs (chicken broiled on a spit with tomatoes, onions and peppers), or a Greek salad.

Avoid: Dishes with large amounts of butter or oil, such as baba ghanouj (eggplant appetizer) and baklava (dessert made with phyllo dough, butter, nuts and honey). To limit sodium, avoid olives, anchovies and feta cheese.

Italian

Look for: Marinara (tomatoes with garlic and onions), Marsala (based in wine), clam sauce and pasta primavera with fresh vegetables and a small amount of oil. Simply prepared fish and chicken dishes are also good choices.

Avoid: Pasta stuffed with cheese or fatty meat and dishes with cream or butter sauces. Veal scaloppine and parmigiana (cooked with Parmesan cheese) contain added fat.

Japanese

Look for: Steamed rice, soba or udon noodles, yakisoba (stir-fried noodles), yakitori (chicken teriyaki), shumai (steamed dumplings), tofu, sukiyaki, kayaku gohan (vegetables and rice).

Avoid: Shrimp or vegetable tempura, chicken katsu, tonkatsu (fried pork), shrimp agemono, fried tofu (bean curd).

Mexican

Look for: Grilled fish, shrimp and chicken with salsa made of tomato, chilies and onion. Order corn tortillas (they're lower in fat and calories than are flour tortillas) as long as they aren't deep-fried. For a side dish, order rice or beans (black, pinto, refried). Make sure your side dishes aren't cooked with fat or lard — ask your server about this.

Avoid: Dishes with large amounts of cheese, sour cream and guacamole. Chips also can add a lot of fat and calories.

How To Avoid Cheat Days On A Dr. Now Diet

Give yourself permission by planning one day a week to eat the desserts you love. By doing this, you will not feel guilt or shame in your mind. Keep plenty of healthy food in your kitchen. By doing this, you avoid eating dessert in half. If you have a must-have item in your home for a special occasion, keep it out of sight. Plan how many calories you are eating each day. Tell people around you that I am losing weight and changing my eating habits. By doing this, all those people will remind you when you are wrong.

Be consistent with your meal times. Start your day with a balanced breakfast. Don't skip meals. Consistent timing gives you control over yourself. Start a Food Journal. By journaling the food you eat, you will notice how much you are eating and when you eat more. Make your body healthy habits. Avoiding sugary drinks is a healthy habit. It is also a good habit to exercise daily to keep your body healthy.

When you eat a meal, there is a conversation going on between your brain and stomach. It takes 20-25 minutes for your brain to know that you are full. Some people finish their meal within 10 minutes then their brain doesn't know if their stomach is full or not so they tend to overeat resulting in weight gain over time.

Dr. Now 30 Days Meal Plan

WEEK 1 MEAL PLAN

MONDAY
Breakfast: Mushroom Omelet
Lunch: American Cobb Egg Salad in Lettuce Wraps
Dinner: CRISPY THIGHS & MASH
Per Day
Calories: 1040; Fat: 72g; Protein: 79g; Net Carbs: 15g

TUESDAY
Breakfast: Breakfast Bowl
Lunch: Feta Bacon Green Salad
Dinner: NOODLES & GLAZED SALMON
Per Day
Calories: 1125; Fat: 79g; Protein: 76g; Net Carbs: 16g

WEDNESDAY
Breakfast: Breakfast Cauliflower Mix
Lunch: Tofu & Spinach Zucchini Lasagna
Dinner: SCALLOPS & MOZZA BROCCOLI MASH
Per Day
Calories: 1007; Fat: 73g; Protein: 77g; Net Carbs: 17g

THURSDAY
Breakfast: Bell Peppers and Avocado Bowls
Lunch: Strawberry & Spinach Blue Cheese Salad
Dinner: BBQ BEEF & SLAW
Per Day
Calories: 1137; Fat: 73g; Protein: 79g; Net Carbs: 20g

FRIDAY
Breakfast: Ham & Cheese Sandwiches
Lunch: Pancetta Mashed Cauliflower
Dinner: CREAM OF MUSHROOM–STUFFED CHICKEN
Per Day
Calories: 1035; Fat: 74g; Protein: 85g; Net Carbs: 14g

SATURDAY
Breakfast: Avocados Stuffed With Salmon
Lunch: Fish Taco Green Bowl with Red Cabbage
Dinner: PORK CHOPS
Per Day
Calories: 1133; Fat: 77g; Protein: 81g; Net Carbs: 14g

SUNDAY
Breakfast: Scrambled Eggs

Lunch: Seitan Kabobs with BBQ Sauce
Dinner: PORK HOCK
Per Day
Calories: 1056; Fat: 76g; Protein: 79g; Net Carbs: 14g

WEEK 2 MEAL PLAN

MONDAY
Breakfast: Nutritious Breakfast Salad
Lunch: Grilled Lamb Chops with Minty Sauce
Dinner: MEATBALLS WITH BACON AND CHEESE
Per Day
Calories: 1002; Fat: 88; Protein: 59g; Net Carbs: 19g

TUESDAY
Breakfast: Berry Hemp Seed Breakfast
Lunch: Burritos with Avocado Greek Yogurt Filling
Dinner: BACON WRAPPED CHICKEN
Per Day
Calories: 975; Fat: 79g; Protein: 87g; Net Carbs: 16g

WEDNESDAY
Breakfast: Morning Chia Pudding
Lunch: Easy Lamb Kebabs
Dinner: SAUSAGE & CABBAGE SKILLET MELT
Per Day
Calories: 1008; Fat: 72g; Protein: 77g; Net Carbs: 22g

THURSDAY
Breakfast: Broccoli, Egg & Pancetta Gratin
Lunch: Cheese Brussels Sprouts Salad
Dinner: SPAGHETTI SQUASH WITH MEAT SAUCE
Per Day
Calories: 1037; Fat: 77g; Protein: 79g; Net Carbs: 20g

FRIDAY
Breakfast: French Toast with Berry Yogurt
Lunch: Prosciutto-Wrapped Chicken with Asparagus
Dinner: CHEESY BACON BRUSSELS SPROUTS
Per Day
Calories: 978; Fat: 78g; Protein: 85g; Net Carbs: 14g

SATURDAY
Breakfast: Breadless Breakfast Sandwich
Lunch: Spinach & Cheese Stuffed Flank Steak Rolls
Dinner: PARMESAN CHICKEN
Per Day
Calories: 1133; Fat: 77g; Protein: 81g; Net Carbs: 14g

SUNDAY
Breakfast: Rolled Smoked Salmon with Avocado
Lunch: Turnip Chips with Avocado Dip
Dinner: CREAMY CHICKEN
Per Day
Calories: 1112; Fat: 73g; Protein: 79g; Net Carbs: 14g

WEEK 3 MEAL PLAN

MONDAY
Breakfast: Breakfast Pork Bagel
Lunch: Classic Egg Salad with Olives
Dinner: LOW CARB CHICKEN NUGGETS
Per Day
Calories: 1140; Fat: 72g; Protein: 79g; Net Carbs: 25g

TUESDAY
Breakfast: Spinach Nests with Eggs & Cheese
Lunch: Chicken Salad with Parmesan
Dinner: TOTCHOS
Per Day
Calories: 1125; Fat: 79g; Protein: 72g; Net Carbs: 16g

WEDNESDAY
Breakfast: Bacon & Mushroom "Tacos"
Lunch: Kale & Broccoli Slaw with Bacon & Parmesan
Dinner: PORK PIES
Per Day
Calories: 1107; Fat: 73g; Protein: 77g; Net Carbs: 17g

THURSDAY
Breakfast: Mushroom & Cheese Lettuce Cups
Lunch: Turkey Bacon & Turnip Salad
Dinner: GLAZED SALMON
Per Day
Calories: 1137; Fat: 77g; Protein: 79g; Net Carbs: 20g

FRIDAY
Breakfast: Tomato and Eggs Salad
Lunch: Chicken, Avocado & Egg Bowls
Dinner: COCONUT SHRIMP
Per Day
Calories: 1135; Fat: 74g; Protein: 80g; Net Carbs: 14g

SATURDAY
Breakfast: Tuna & Egg Salad with Chili Mayo
Lunch: Spinach Salad with Pancetta & Mustard

Dinner: Cheesy Eggplant Casserole
Per Day
Calories: 1133; Fat: 77g; Protein: 81g; Net Carbs: 14g

SUNDAY
Breakfast: Avocado Shakshuka
Lunch: Modern Greek Salad with Avocado
Dinner: Spinach & Mushroom Casserole
Per Day
Calories: 1112; Fat: 74g; Protein: 79g; Net Carbs: 14g

WEEK 4 MEAL PLAN

MONDAY
Breakfast: Lazy Eggs with Feta Cheese
Lunch: Cheesy Beef Salad
Dinner: Beef & Spinach Casserole
Per Day
Calories: 1140; Fat: 72g; Protein: 79g; Net Carbs: 25g

TUESDAY
Breakfast: Seasoned Hard Boiled Eggs
Lunch: Chicken Salad with Gorgonzola Cheese
Dinner: Taco Soup
Per Day
Calories: 1108; Fat: 76g; Protein: 68g; Net Carbs: 16g

WEDNESDAY
Breakfast: Deli Ham Eggs
Lunch: Cheddar & Turkey Meatball Salad
Dinner: Bacon & Zucchini Casserole
Per Day
Calories: 1107; Fat: 33g; Protein: 77g; Net Carbs: 17g

THURSDAY
Breakfast: Goat Cheese Frittata with Asparagus
Lunch: Shrimp Salad with Avocado
Dinner: Chicken & Artichoke Casserole
Per Day
Calories: 1148; Fat: 69g; Protein: 79g; Net Carbs: 20g

FRIDAY
Breakfast: Shrimp and Bacon Breakfast
Lunch: Green Salad with Feta & Blueberries
Dinner: Chicken Curry Casserole
Per Day
Calories: 1135; Fat: 74g; Protein: 85g; Net Carbs: 14g

SATURDAY
Breakfast: Beef, Avocado and Eggs
Lunch: Easy Beef Stroganoff
Dinner: Asparagus Stuffed Chicken Breasts
Per Day
Calories: 1033; Fat: 67g; Protein: 81g; Net Carbs: 14g

SUNDAY
Breakfast: Pork and Avocado Mix
Lunch: Beef Teriyaki with Chinese Cabbage
Dinner: Celery & Grouper Casserole
Per Day
Calories: 998; Fat: 73g; Protein: 79g; Net Carbs: 14g

Recipes For Meal Plan

Breakfast

1.Mushroom Omelet

Ingredients for 4 servings:
2 spring onions, chopped
½ pound white mushrooms
Salt and black pepper to the taste
4 eggs, whisked
1 tablespoon olive oil
½ teaspoon cumin, ground
1 tablespoon cilantro, chopped

Instructions: (10 minutes preparation time, 20 minutes cooking time):

Take one pan and set it on medium temperature. Add spring, onions and mushrooms to it. Let this mixture cook for 5 minutes. Add eggs to it, after mixing gently, cover and cook on medium flame for 15 minutes. Cut the omelet into pieces and serve on a plate for breakfast.

Nutrition: calories 109, fat 8.1, fiber 0.8, carbs 2.9, protein 7.5

2.Breakfast Bowl

Preparation time: 10 minutes
Cooking time: 20 minutes
Servings: 1

Ingredients:

4 ounces ground beef
1 onion, peeled and chopped
8 mushrooms, sliced
Salt and ground black pepper, to taste
2 eggs, whisked
1 tablespoon coconut oil
½ teaspoon smoked paprika
1 avocado, pitted, peeled, and chopped
12 black olives, pitted and sliced

Directions:

Take oil in a pan and heat it on medium flame. Add mushrooms, onions, salt and pepper to it. Stir the mixture well and let it cook for 5 minutes. Add paprika and beef. Stir well and cook for 10 minutes. Take it in a bowl and shake it well. Take the pan and heat it again on medium heat. Add eggs, little salt, pepper and scramble. Add the beef mixture back to the pan and mix. Add the olives and avocado and cook for 1 minute. Take the mixture in a bowl and mix and serve.

Nutrition: Calories – 1002, Fat – 74,9, Fiber – 19,4, Carbs – 36,9, Protein – 55,6

3.Breakfast Cauliflower Mix

Preparation time: 10 minutes
Cooking time: 25 minutes
Servings: 4

Ingredients:

2 tablespoons ghee
1 small yellow onion, chopped
2 garlic cloves, minced
3 jalapeno peppers, chopped
1 pound beef meat, lean and ground
A pinch of salt and black pepper
1 cauliflower head, grated
½ cup water
½ cup homemade mayonnaise
¼ cup sunflower seed butter
1 teaspoon cumin, ground
1 tablespoons coconut aminos
4 eggs
½ avocado, peeled, cored and chopped
1 tablespoon parsley, chopped

Directions:

Take a pan and heat it on medium flame. Heat ghee in it. Add the onions, jalapeño and garlic. and cook for 3 minutes. Add meat, salt and pepper. Stir the mixture well and cook for another 5 minutes. Add sunflower seed butter, aminos, water, mayo, cumin. Mix and cook for another 5 minutes. Make 4 holes in this mixture. Crack an egg into each hole and sprinkle with pepper and salt. Then put this mixture in preheated oven and cook for 10 minutes. Divide the mixture between plates and add avocado slices to serve.

Nutrition: calories 288, fat 12, fiber 6, carbs 15, protein 38

4. Bell Peppers and Avocado Bowls

Ingredients for 4 servings:

2 tablespoons olive oil   2 shallots, chopped
1 red bell pepper, cut into strips
1 yellow bell pepper, cut into strips
1 green bell pepper, cut into strips
1 big avocado, peeled, pitted, and cut into wedges
1 teaspoon sweet paprika
½ cup vegetable stock
Salt and black pepper to the taste
1 tablespoon chives, chopped

Instructions: (10 minutes preparation time, 15 minutes cooking time):

Take oil in a pan and heat it on medium flame. Add peanuts and saute for 2 minutes. Add avocado, bell pepper and other ingredients. Bring to a boil and cook on medium heat for another 10 minutes. Mix the chives and divide between plates and serve for breakfast.

Nutrition: calories 194, fat 17.1, fiber 4.9, carbs 11.5, protein 2

5.Ham & Cheese Sandwiches

Ingredients for 2 servings

4 eggs
½ tsp baking powder
5 tbsp butter, softened
4 tbsp almond flour
2 tbsp psyllium husk powder
2 slices mozzarella cheese
2 slices smoked ham

Directions and Total Time: approx. 20 minutes

For making buns, mix baking powder, almond flour, 4 tbsp butter, eggs and bran powder in a bowl. Mix until a dough is formed. Place the batter in two ovenproof mugs and microwave for 2 minutes to set. Then remove the buns, flip them over and let them cool, then cut them in half. Place a slice of hamcha and a slice of mozzarella cheese on a bun. And then put the second banavar. Heat remaining butter in a pan. Grill the sandwich until the cheese melts and then serve.

Per serving: Cal 616; Net Carbs 4g; Fat 55g; Protein 30g

6.Avocados Stuffed With Salmon

Preparation time: 10 minutes
Cooking time: 0 minutes
Servings: 2
Ingredients:
1 big avocado, pitted and halved
2 ounces smoked salmon, flaked
Juice of 1 lemon
2 tablespoons olive oil
1 ounce goat cheese, crumbled
A pinch of salt and black pepper

Directions:

Take a food processor and mix salmon, oil, lemon juice, salt and pepper in it. Divide the mixture in half from the avocado halves and serve.

Nutrition: calories 300m fat 15, fiber 5, carbs 8, protein 16

7.Scrambled Eggs

Preparation time: 10 minutes
Cooking time: 10 minutes
Servings: 1

Ingredients:

4 bell mushrooms, chopped
3 eggs, whisked
Salt and ground black pepper, to taste
2 ham slices, chopped
¼ cup red bell pepper, seeded and chopped
½ cup spinach, chopped
1 tablespoon coconut oil

Directions:

Take half the oil in a pan and heat it on medium flame. Add bell pepper, spinach, mushroom and baken and cook for 5 minutes. Heat another pan with remaining oil on medium heat, add eggs and scramble. Add pepper, vegetables, salt and ham and mix well. Cook for a minute and serve.

Nutrition: Calories – 430, Fat – 31,9, Fiber – 2,4, Carbs – 9, Protein – 29,5

8.Nutritious Breakfast Salad

Preparation time: 10 minutes
Cooking time: 6 minutes
Servings: 2

Ingredients:

3 cups kale, torn
1 teaspoon red vinegar
A pinch of salt and black pepper
2 teaspoons olive oil
2 eggs
4 strips bacon, chopped
10 cherry tomatoes, halved
2 ounces avocado, pitted, peeled and sliced

Directions:

Take some water in a bowl. Bring to a boil over medium heat. Add eggs to it and let it boil for 5 minutes. Then drain the water. Wash, peel, cut and cool the eggs. In a bowl, mix eggs, tomatoes, oil, baken, avocado, salt, pepper and black vinegar. Divide between salad plates and serve for breakfast.

Nutrition: calories 292, fat 14, fiber 7, carbs 18, protein 16

9.Berry Hemp Seed Breakfast

Ingredients for 2 servings

½ cup berry medley
1 cup coconut milk
¼ tsp vanilla extract
4 oz heavy cream
2 tbsp hemp seeds
4 tsp liquid stevia
1 tbsp sugar-free maple syrup

Directions and Total Time: approx. 10 min + cooling time

Place berries in a medium bowl and mash with a fork until pureed. Add liquid stevia, heavy cream vanilla, vanilla, coconut milk and hemp. Mix well and refrigerate overnight. Serve pudding in serving glasses then garnish with maple syrup.

Per serving: Cal 532; Net Carbs 7g; Fat 46g; Protein 10g

10.Morning Chia Pudding

Ingredients for 2 servings

2 tbsp chia seeds
¾ cup coconut milk
1 tbsp chopped walnuts
½ tsp vanilla extract
½ cup blueberries

Directions and Total Time: approx. 10 min + chilling time

Place half of the blueberries, coconut milk, and vanilla in a blender. Mix until the blueberries are well mixed. Add chia seeds to that mixture. Divide the mixture between two bowls and keep it covered in the refrigerator for 4 hours. Serve with black walnuts and blueberries to allow it to gel.

Per serving: Cal 299; Net Carbs 7g; Fat 28g; Protein 9g

11.Broccoli, Egg & Pancetta Gratin

Ingredients for 2 servings

10 oz broccoli florets
1 red bell pepper, chopped
4 slices pancetta, chopped
2 tsp olive oil
1 tsp dried oregano
Salt and black pepper to taste
4 fresh eggs
4 tbsp Parmesan cheese

Directions and Total Time: approx. 30 minutes

Preheat the oven to 420 F. Line a baking sheet with wax paper. Take a pan and heat olive oil in it on medium heat. Saute the pancetta in that pan for 4 minutes. Take a baking sheet and place pancetta, broccoli, bell pepper on it and stir together. Add salt, oregano and pepper to it. Let the vegetables cook until soft. Make four indentations and add the egg. Then sprinkle parmesan cheese over it and cook in the oven for 5 to 7 minutes and then serve.

Per serving: Cal 464; Net Carbs 8.2g; Fat 30g; Protein 30g

12.French Toast With Berry Yogurt

Ingredients for 2 servings
½ cup strawberries, halved

½ cup raspberries
2 eggs
1 cup Greek yogurt
2 tbsp sugar-free maple syrup
¼ tsp cinnamon powder
¼ tsp nutmeg powder
2 tbsp almond milk
4 zero-carb bread slices
1 ½ tbsp butter
1 tbsp olive oil

Directions and Total Time: approx. 20 min + chilling time

Take a bowl and mix maple syrup, berries and curd in it. Allow the mixture to cool for an hour. Take another bowl and whisk eggs, cinnamon, nutmeg and almond milk in it. Keep this bowl aside. Cut the bread into 4 pieces. Take a pan and heat olive oil and butter on medium heat. Dip each slice of bread into the egg mixture and bake for 5 to 7 minutes until both sides are crispy. Serve hot with berries and yogurt.

Per serving: Cal 401; Net Carbs 9g; Fat 26g; Protein 17g

13.Breadless Breakfast Sandwich

Preparation time: 10 minutes
Cooking time: 10 minutes
Servings: 1

Ingredients:
2 eggs
Salt and ground black pepper, to taste
2 tablespoons butter
¼ pound pork sausage, minced
¼ cup water
1 tablespoon guacamole

Directions:

Take a bowl and mix pepper, minced sausage meat and a pinch of salt in it and mix well. Make patties out of this mix. Take a pan and heat a tablespoon of butter in it on medium heat. Add sausage patty to it and fry for 4 minutes on each side. Break an egg into two bowls, add spices and salt and whisk. Heat a pan with the remaining butter over medium heat. Place two heated biscuit cutters in the pan. And put an egg in each. Add water and reduce the heat. Cover the pan for 4 minutes to cook the eggs. Transfer the egg buns to a paper towel to drain all the grease. Place sausage patty on egg bun, spread guacamole on top. And then cover the bun with the second egg.

Nutritional Value: Calories – 735, Fat – 66, Fiber – 0.5, Carbs – 1.7, Protein – 33.6

14. Rolled Smoked Salmon with Avocado

Ingredients for 2 servings

2 tbsp cream cheese, softened
1 lime, zested and juiced
½ avocado, pitted, peeled
1 tbsp mint, chopped
Salt to taste
2 slices smoked salmon

Directions and Total Time: approx. 10 min + cooling time

Take a bowl and smash the avocado in it using a fork. Add mint, salt, cream cheese lime, and juice and mix well. Fill each piece of salmon with the cream cheese mix and place in a piece of wrap. Roll the salmon into a ball, twist and secure the ends. Then keep it in the refrigerator for 2 hours. Remove the plastic and cut off the wraps at both ends. Then cut the rolls into 1/2 inch pieces and serve.

Per serving: Cal 520; Net Carbs 3g; Fat 31g; Protein 50g

15. Breakfast Pork Bagel

Preparation time: 10 minutes
Cooking time: 40 minutes
Servings: 6

Ingredients:

1 yellow onion, chopped
1 tablespoon ghee
2 pounds pork meat, ground
2 eggs
2/3 cup tomato sauce
A pinch of salt and black pepper
1 teaspoon sweet paprika

Directions:

Take a pan, take ghee in it and heat it on medium flame. Add onion and cook for 5 minutes. Then take a big pot and mix the meat, tomato sauce, salt, pepper, fried onions and paprika in it. Mix well and make 6 bagls with your hand. Divide bagels among plates and serve for breakfast.

Nutrition: calories 300, fat 11, fiber 8, carbs 16, protein 12

16.Spinach Nests with Eggs & Cheese

Ingredients for 2 servings

1 tbsp olive oil
1 tbsp dried dill
1 lb spinach, chopped
1 tbsp pine nuts
Salt and black pepper to taste
¼ cup feta cheese, crumbled
2 eggs

Directions and Total Time: approx. 30 minutes

Take olive oil in a pan and saute spinach in it on medium temperature. Sprinkle salt and pepper and keep aside. Take a baking sheet and coat it with cooking spray. Make two spinach nests on a baking sheet and crack an egg into each nest. Sprinkle with dill and garnish with feta. Bake at 350 F for 20 minutes until the egg whites are set and the yolk is still runny. Serve the nest on a plate garnished with pine nuts.

Per serving: Cal 308; Net Carbs 5.4g; Fat 22g; Protein 18g

17.Bacon & Mushroom "Tacos"

Ingredients for 2 servings

1 egg, hard-boiled and chopped
1 cup mushrooms, sliced
3 oz mozzarella cheese, grated
3 oz bacon, chopped
1 shallot, sliced
1 avocado, sliced
1 tbsp salsa
1 tbsp sour cream

Directions and Total Time: approx. 30 minutes

First preheat the oven to 350 F. Set 2 piles of mozzarella cheese on a parchment-lined oven dish. Gently set with your hands to form taco shells. Bake in the oven for 10 minutes, take out and let cool. Take a skillet over medium heat and cook the bacon for 5 minutes until crisp and transfer to an oven safe dish. Saute the mushrooms and shallots in the same grease. Move away from bacon. Mix the eggs. Divide mixture among taco shells and serve with salsa, avocado and sour cream.

Per serving: Cal 563; Net Carbs 8g; Fat 48g; Protein 22g

18.Mushroom & Cheese Lettuce Cups

Ingredients for 2 servings

1 tbsp olive oil
½ onion, chopped
Salt and black pepper to taste
½ cup mushrooms, chopped
¼ tsp cayenne pepper
2 fresh lettuce leaves
2 slices Gruyere cheese
1 tomato, sliced

Directions and Total Time: approx. 20 minutes

Take olive oil in a pan and heat it on medium heat. Fry the onion in it for 4 minutes and cook for 4 minutes. Add mushroom and red chilli to it and cook for 5 minutes. Add salt and pepper to taste. Add the mushroom mixture to the lettuce leaves and serve topped with cheese and tomato slices.

Per serving: Cal 281; Net Carbs 5.7g; Fat 22g; Protein 12g

19.Tomato and Eggs Salad

Ingredients for 4 servings:

4 eggs, hard boiled, peeled and cut into wedges
2 cups cherry tomatoes, halved
1 cup kalamata olives, pitted and halved
1 cup baby arugula
2 spring onions, chopped
A pinch of salt and black pepper
1 tablespoon avocado oil

Instructions: (5 minutes preparation time, 0 minutes cooking time):

Take a bowl and mix eggs, tomatoes and other ingredients in it. Toss and serve in small bowls.

Nutrition: calories 126, fat 8.6, fiber 2.6, carbs 6.9, protein 6.9

20.Tuna & Egg Salad with Chili Mayo

Ingredients for 4 servings

4 eggs
14 oz tuna in brine, drained
½ small head lettuce, torn

2 spring onions, chopped
¼ cup ricotta, crumbled
2 tbsp sour cream
½ tbsp mustard powder
½ cup mayonnaise
½ tbsp lemon juice
½ tbsp chili powder
2 dill pickles, sliced
Salt and black pepper to taste

Directions and Total Time: approx. 20 minutes

Boil eggs in salted water on medium heat for 10 minutes. Allow them to cool on an ice bath. Then cut it into small pieces. Take the pieces in a bowl. Add tuna, mustard powder and onions. Then add sour cream, ricotta and lettuce. Take a bowl and mix egg yolk, lemon juice and chili powder in it. Mix to your liking. Serve with pickles.

Per serving: Cal 391; Net Carbs 4.5g; Fat 22g; Protein 35g

21.Avocado Shakshuka

Ingredients for 2 servings

4 eggs
1 avocado, chopped
1 tbsp olive oil
1 medium red onion, sliced
1 zucchini, sliced
1 red bell pepper, sliced
1 yellow bell pepper, sliced
1 medium tomato, diced
1 cup vegetable broth
1 tbsp chopped parsley

Directions and Total Time: approx. 25 minutes

Heat olive oil in a pan. Add onions, zucchini and bell pepper to it and fry for 10 minutes. Add the mutton and tomato stock. Bring to a boil then reduce heat until thickened. Make four holes in the sauce and put eggs in it. Let the eggs boil and turn off the heat. Add avocado and eggs and serve hot.

Per serving: Cal 448; Net Carbs 10g; Fat 39g; Protein 18g

22.Lazy Eggs with Feta Cheese

Ingredients for 2 servings

4 eggs
¼ cup coconut milk
¼ cup feta cheese, grated
1 garlic clove, minced
¼ tsp dried dill
¼ tsp red pepper flakes

Directions and Total Time: approx. 10 minutes

Take a bowl and beat the egg lightly using a fork. Add the flakes, coconut milk and feta garlic. Divide this mixture into microwave safe cups. Leave the microwave on for 45 minutes. Then mix and keep in the microwave for another 75 minutes. Serve sprinkled with dill.

Per serving: Cal 234; Net Carbs 2.7g; Fat 16g; Protein 17g

23.Seasoned Hard Boiled Eggs

Preparation time: 10 minutes
Cooking time: 4 minutes
Servings: 12

Ingredients:

4 tea bags
4 tablespoons salt
12 eggs
2 tablespoons ground cinnamon
6 star anise
1 teaspoon ground black pepper
1 tablespoon peppercorns
8 cups water
1 cup tamari sauce

Directions:

Take a pot, add water and boil eggs on medium temperature. Cook till it becomes hard. Once they are cool, break them without peeling them. Prepare a mixture of water, salt, pepper, tea bags, cinnamon, pepper, star anise, tamari sauce in a large saucepan. Add the beaten eggs to it, cover the pot and simmer on low for 30 minutes. Remove the tea bags and boil the eggs for three and a half hours. Peel the eggs and serve after cooling.

Nutrition: Calories – 122, Fat – 4.6, Fiber – 0.8, Carbs – 6.7, Protein – 13.9

24.Deli Ham Eggs

Ingredients for 2 servings

2 tbsp butter
1 shallot, chopped
Salt and black pepper to taste
2 slices deli ham, chopped
4 eggs
1 thyme sprig, chopped
½ cup olives, pitted and sliced

Directions and Total Time: approx. 20 minutes

In a bowl, gently beat the eggs with a fork. Keep the heat on medium and then set the skillet with the hot butter. Sauté for 5 minutes until soft. Add ham, pepper and salt. After cooking for 5 minutes, garnish with olives and serve.

Per serving: Cal 431; Net Carbs 6g; Fat 36g; Protein 21g

25.Goat Cheese Frittata with Asparagus

Ingredients for 2 servings

1 tbsp olive oil
½ onion, chopped
1 cup asparagus, chopped
4 eggs, beaten
½ habanero pepper, minced
Salt and red pepper, to taste
¾ cup goat cheese, crumbled
1 tbsp parsley, chopped

Directions and Total Time: approx. 35 minutes

Preheat the oven to 350 F. Saute onion in olive oil for about 10 minutes until caramelized. Add Shatavari to the pan and boil until soft. Add the habaneros and eggs. Add salt and cayenne to your liking. Cook until eggs are cooked. Sprinkle the goat cheese and eggs over the frittata. Cook in the oven for 25 minutes and serve.

Per serving: Cal 345; Net Carbs 8.3g; Fat 37g; Protein 32g

26.Shrimp and Bacon Breakfast

Preparation time: 10 minutes

Cooking time: 15 minutes
Servings: 4

Ingredients:

1 cup mushrooms, sliced
4 bacon slices, chopped
4 ounces smoked salmon, chopped
4 ounces shrimp, deveined
Salt and ground black pepper, to taste
½ cup coconut cream

Directions:

Take a pan and heat it on medium heat, add bacon and cook for 5 minutes. Add the mushrooms and cook, stirring for 5 minutes, then simmer for 5 minutes. Add salmon, stir and cook for 4 minutes. Add prawns and cook for 2 minutes. Sprinkle it with salt, coconut cream and pepper. Cook well for 1 minute and serve.

Nutrition: Calories – 242, Fat – 16.8, Fiber – 0.8, Carbs – 2.9, Protein – 19.9

27.Beef, Avocado and Eggs

Preparation time: 10 minutes
Cooking time: 11 minutes
Servings: 2

Ingredients:

8 mushrooms, sliced
1 yellow onion, chopped
1 tablespoon olive oil
3 ounces beef, ground
A pinch of salt and black pepper
2 eggs, whisked
½ teaspoon smoked paprika
1 avocado, peeled, pitted and chopped
10 black olives, pitted and sliced

Directions:

Heat a pan on medium heat. And add beef to it. Stir and cook for 5 minutes. Add mushroom, onion and stir and cook for another 3-4 minutes. Add salt, paprika, pepper and eggs and toss in the oven for another 3-4 minutes. Then divide between bowls and serve with olives and avocado in each bowl.

Nutrition: calories 251, fat 4, fiber 8, carbs 14, protein 6

28. Pork and Avocado Mix

Ingredients for 4 servings:

½ cup tomato passata   1 pound pork, ground
1 avocado, peeled, pitted, and roughly cubed
1 tomato, cubed
Salt and black pepper to the taste
8 eggs, whisked
2 spring onions, chopped
1 tablespoon avocado oil
½ teaspoon cayenne pepper
1 tablespoon chives, chopped

Instructions: (10 minutes preparation time, 22 minutes cooking time):

Take a pan and heat it with oil on medium flame. Add spring onions to it. Let it cook well for 1-2 minutes. Add red pepper, tomatoes and meat. Let it cook for another 5-6 minutes. Add tomato paste, avocado, egg, pepper and salt to it. Toss and cook on medium heat for another 15-20 minutes. Divide into bowls and serve as breakfast.

Nutrition: calories 431, fat 26.1, fiber 4.1, carbs 6.8, protein 42.3

29. Turkey Breakfast

Preparation time: 10 minute
Cooking time: 20 minutes
Servings: 1

Ingredients:
2 avocado slices
Salt and ground black pepper, to taste
2 bacon slices, diced
2 turkey breast slices, already cooked
2 tablespoons coconut oil
2 eggs, whisked

Directions:

Heat a pan over medium heat and add the bacon pieces. Cook it. Take another pan and add oil to it and heat it on medium temperature. Add salt, egg and pepper to it and scramble. Serve for breakfast with turkey breast bacon slices, scrambled eggs, bacon and avocado slices on two plates.

Nutritional Value: Calories – 791, Fat – 64.3, Fiber – 5.4, Carbs – 11.8, Protein – 41.8

30.Mexican Breakfast

Preparation time: 10 minutes
Cooking time: 30 minutes
Servings: 8

Ingredients:

½ cup tomato paste
½ tsp garlic powder
1 tsp dried basil
1 tsp dried oregano
1 tsp cumin
2 tsp chili powder
1 pound ground pork
1 pound chorizo, chopped
Salt and ground black pepper, to taste
8 eggs
1 tomato, cored and chopped
3 tablespoons butter
½ cup onion, chopped
1 avocado, pitted, peeled, and chopped

Directions:

Take a bowl and mix tomato paste and spices for enchilada sauce. In another bowl, mix the pork and chorizo. Mix well and place on a baking sheet. Drizzle enchilada sauce over it. Then place at 350 F. Then wait 20 minutes to bake. Take a pan, melt butter on medium heat, add eggs and then scramble. Remove the pork mixture from the oven and spread the scrambled egg mixture over the top. Sprinkle salt, tomato, avocado, pepper and onion on it. Then divide into plates and serve.

Nutrition: Calories – 513, Fat – 37.6, Fiber – 2.8, Carbs – 8.4, Protein – 35.6

Lunch

1.American Cobb Egg Salad in Lettuce Wraps

Ingredients for 4 servings
2 chicken breasts, cubed
1 tbsp olive oil
6 large eggs
2 tomatoes, seeded, chopped
6 tbsp cream cheese
1 head lettuce, leaves separated

Directions and Total Time: approx. 30 minutes

Preheat the oven to 400 F. Place the chicken pieces in a bowl, drizzle with olive oil and sprinkle with salt and pepper. Mix until the chicken is well coated. Place the chicken on a greased baking sheet. Bake for 8 minutes, turning once. Boil eggs in salted water for 10 minutes. Peel the eggs by running them under cold water. And cut into small pieces. Take the salad in a bowl. Remove chicken from oven and add to salad bowl. Add cream cheese and tomatoes to it. Add 2 lettuce leaves each as a cup. and top each with 2 tablespoons of egg salad and serve.

Per serving: Cal 325; Net Carbs 4g; Fat 24.5g; Protein 21g

2.Feta Bacon Green Salad

Ingredients for 4 servings
2 (8 oz) pack mixed salad greens
1 ½ cups feta cheese, crumbled
8 strips bacon
1 tbsp white wine vinegar
3 tbsp extra virgin olive oil
Salt and black pepper to taste

Directions and Total Time: approx. 20 minutes

Take a bowl and add all the green vegetables in it. and keep aside. Fry the bacon strips in a pan for 5-6 minutes until crisp. Chop it and spread it on the salad. Toss with half the cheese and set aside. Take a small bowl and whisk together the salt, olive oil, white vinegar, and black pepper until well combined. Toss and serve with remaining cheese.

Per serving: Cal 205; Net Carbs 2g; Fat 20g; Protein 4g

3.Tofu & Spinach Zucchini Lasagna

Ingredients for 4 servings

2 zucchinis, sliced
Salt and black pepper to taste
2 cups cream cheese
2 cups tofu cheese, shredded
3 cups tomato sauce
1 cup packed baby spinach

Directions and Total Time: approx. 60 minutes

Preheat the oven to 370 F. Mix tofu, black pepper, salt, cream cheese evenly. Spread 1/4 cup of the mixture in the bottom of a greased baking dish. Top with 1/3 of the zucchini slices. Spread 1 cup tomato sauce. And spread a third of the spinach on top. Repeat this layering process twice. Grease one end of the foil with cooking spray and cover the baking dish with foil. Bake for 40 minutes, remove the foil and bake for another 15 minutes. Let sit for 5-6 minutes, slice and serve.

Per serving: Cal 390; Net Carbs 2g; Fat 39g; Protein 7g

4.Strawberry & Spinach Blue Cheese Salad

Ingredients for 2 servings

1 ½ cups gorgonzola cheese, grated
4 cups spinach
4 strawberries, sliced
½ cup flaked almonds
4 tbsp raspberry vinaigrette

Directions and Total Time: approx. 20 minutes

Preheat the oven to 400 F. Spread Gorgonzola cheese on 2 pieces of parchment paper. And bake for 10-12 minutes. Take 2 similar bowls and place them upside down and place 2 pieces of parchment paper on top to give the cheese a bowl shape. Let cool for 10 minutes. Mix the spinach in these bowls. Drizzle with vinaigrette. Top with almonds and strawberries and serve.

Per serving: Cal 445; Net Carbs: 5.3g; Fat: 34g; Protein: 33g

5.Pancetta Mashed Cauliflower

Ingredients for 6 servings

3 heads cauliflower, leaves removed
6 slices pancetta
2 cups water
2 tbsp melted butter
½ cup buttermilk
¼ cup Colby cheese, grated
2 tbsp chopped chives

Directions and Total Time: approx. 40 minutes

Preheat the oven to 350 F. Heat a pan and fry the pancetta for 5 minutes. Allow to cool and crumble. Keep the pancetta fat. Take a pot and boil the cauliflower head in it for 10 minutes. Remove and keep in a bowl. Add buttermilk, butter, pepper, salt and puree until smooth. Grease a casserole dish with pancetta fat. And spread the mash in it. Sprinkle with Colby cheese. Place under broiler for 5 minutes. Serve with chopped chives.

Per serving: Cal 312; Net Carbs 6g; Fat 25g; Protein 14g

6.Fish Taco Green Bowl with Red Cabbage

Ingredients for 4 servings

2 cups broccoli, chopped
2 tsp ghee
4 tilapia fillets, cut into cubes
¼ tsp taco seasoning
Salt and chili pepper to taste
¼ head red cabbage, shredded
1 ripe avocado, chopped
1 tsp dill

Directions and Total Time: approx. 20 minutes

Take a bowl, take some water in it and sprinkle the broccoli. Keep in microwave for 5 minutes. Fluff with a fork and set aside. Take a pan, melt ghee in it and rub the tilapia with tako masala, salt, chilli and cumin. And fry until brown. Set aside for 10 minutes, add broccoli, fish, avocado and cabbage to 4 serving bowls and serve.

Per serving: Cal 269; Net Carbs 4g; Fat 23.4g; Protein 16.5g

7.Seitan Kabobs with BBQ Sauce

Ingredients for 4 servings

10 oz seitan, cut into chunks
1 ½ cups water
1 red onion, cut into chunks
1 red bell pepper, cut chunks
1 yellow bell pepper, chopped
2 tbsp olive oil
1 cup barbecue sauce
Salt and black pepper to taste

Directions and Total Time: approx. 2 hours 30 minutes

Boil water in a pan, turn off the heat and add seitan. Cover the pot of water and let it steam. Take a bowl and add barbecue sauce to it. Add seitan to it and coat with sauce. Cover the pot and marinate in the fridge for 2 hours. Preheat grill to 350 F. seitan, onion, yellow bell pepper. Thread the red bell pepper. Brush the grill grates with olive oil. Place skewers on top and brush with barbecue sauce. Cook kabobs for 5 minutes while basting with sauce.

Per serving: Cal 228; Net Carbs 3.6g; Fat 15g; Protein 13.2g

8. Grilled Lamb Chops with Minty Sauce

Ingredients for 4 servings

8 lamb chops
2 tbsp favorite spice mix
¼ cup olive oil
1 tsp red pepper flakes
2 tbsp lemon juice
2 tbsp fresh mint
3 garlic cloves, pressed
2 tbsp lemon zest
¼ cup parsley
½ tsp smoked paprika

Directions and Total Time: approx. 25 minutes

Heat grill to medium temperature. Rub the lamb with oil and sprinkle with spices. Grill for 2-3 minutes on each side. Whisk together remaining oil, cumin, mint, parsley, paprika and lemon juice. Serve the chops with the sauce.

Per serving: Cal 392; Net Carbs 0g; Fat 31g; Protein 29g

9. Burritos with Avocado Greek Yogurt Filling

Ingredients for 4 servings

2 cups cauli rice
6 zero carb flatbread
2 cups Greek yogurt
1 ½ cups tomato herb salsa
2 avocados, sliced

Directions and Total Time: approx. 5 minutes

Take cauli rice in a bowl, sprinkle water on it and soften it in microwave for 3 minutes. Spread Greek yogurt on flatbread and top with salsa. Spread the cauli rice on top and spread the avocado evenly over it. Fold it and cut it into two pieces.

Per serving: Cal 303; Net Carbs 6g; Fat 25g; Protein 8g

10. Easy Lamb Kebabs

Ingredients for 4 servings

1 pound ground lamb
¼ tsp cinnamon
1 egg
1 grated onion
Salt and black pepper to taste
2 tbsp mint, chopped

Directions and Total Time: approx. 20 minutes

Take a bowl and mix all the ingredients in it. Cut the meat into 4 pieces. Shape all parts of the meat. Heat the grill to medium temperature. Heat the kebab for 5 minutes on each side.

Per serving: Cal 467; Net Carbs 3.2g; Fat 37g; Protein 27g

11.Cheese Brussels Sprouts Salad

Ingredients for 6 servings

2 lb Brussels sprouts, halved
3 tbsp olive oil
Salt and black pepper to taste
2 ½ tbsp balsamic vinegar
¼ red cabbage, shredded
1 tbsp Dijon mustard
1 cup Parmesan, grated
2 tbsp pumpkin seeds, toasted

Directions and Total Time: approx. 35 minutes

Preheat oven to 400 F. Line a baking sheet with foil. Take a bowl and toss the Brussels sprouts with olive oil, salt, pepper, balsamic vinegar and spread on a baking sheet. Bake for 30 minutes. Remove the salad to a bowl. Add half the remaining cheese, red cabbage, mustard. Serve sprinkled with pumpkin and remaining cheese.

Per serving: Cal 210; Net Carbs 6g; Fat 18g; Protein 4g

12.Prosciutto-Wrapped Chicken with Asparagus

Ingredients for 4 servings

6 chicken breasts
8 prosciutto slices
4 tbsp olive oil
1 lb asparagus spears

2 tbsp fresh lemon juice
Manchego cheese for topping

Directions and Total Time: approx. 50 minutes

Preheat oven to 400 F. Sprinkle salt and pepper over chicken, wrap 2 prosciutto slices around chicken breast. Bake on a parchment lined baking sheet for 30 minutes. Preheat the grill to medium heat. Brush asparagus spears with olive oil and sprinkle with salt. Grill for 10 minutes, turning until slightly charred. Remove to a plate and add lemon juice over it. Serve with grated Manchego cheese on top.

Per serving: Cal 468; Net Carbs 2g; Fat 38g; Protein 26g

13. Spinach & Cheese Stuffed Flank Steak Rolls

Ingredients for 6 servings

1 ½ lb flank steak
Salt and black pepper to taste
1 cup ricotta cheese, crumbled
½ loose cup baby spinach
1 jalapeño pepper, chopped
¼ cup chopped basil leaves

Directions and Total Time: approx. 45 minutes

Preheat the oven to 400 F. Wrap the steak in plastic. Place it on a flat surface and run the rolling pin to flatten it. Remove the wraps. Sprinkle with jalapeno, basil leaves, spinach and half of the ricotta cheese. Turn the steak over the stuffing and place on a greased baking sheet. Cook for 30 minutes, turning once. After cooling for 5 minutes, cut into pinwheels. And serve with fried vegetables.

Per serving: Cal 490; Net Carbs 2g; Fat 41g; Protein 28g

14. Turnip Chips with Avocado Dip

Ingredients for 6 servings

2 avocados, mashed
2 tsp lime juice
2 garlic cloves, minced
2 tbsp olive oil
For turnip chips
1 ½ pounds turnips, sliced
1 tbsp olive oil
½ tsp onion powder
½ tsp garlic powder

Directions and Total Time: approx. 20 minutes

Stir together the lemon juice, garlic, salt, 2 tablespoons olive oil, pepper, and avocado. Remove to a bowl and set the oven to 300 F. Set the turnip slices on a baking sheet. Toss with salt, garlic powder, and 1 teaspoon olive oil. Bake for 20 minutes and serve with avocado dip.

Per serving: Cal 269; Net Carbs: 9.4g; Fat: 27g; Protein: 3g

15.Classic Egg Salad with Olives

Ingredients for 2 servings

4 eggs
¼ cup mayonnaise
½ tsp sriracha sauce
½ tbsp mustard
¼ cup scallions
¼ stalk celery, minced
Salt and black pepper to taste
1 head romaine lettuce, torn
¼ tsp fresh lime juice
10 black olives

Directions and Total Time: approx. 15 minutes

Take a pot, add egg and little salt and boil it on medium temperature. After cooling, peel the eggs and cut them into small pieces. Take it in a salad bowl and mix it with the rest of the ingredients. Serve with a sprinkle of scallions on top.

Per serving: Cal 442; Net Carbs 9g; Fat 32g; Protein 24g

16.Chicken Salad with Parmesan

Ingredients for 2 servings

½ lb chicken breasts, sliced
¼ cup lemon juice
2 garlic cloves, minced
2 tbsp olive oil
1 romaine lettuce, shredded
3 Parmesan crisps
2 tbsp Parmesan, grated Dressing
2 tbsp extra virgin olive oil
1 tbsp lemon juice

Salt and black pepper to taste

Directions and Total Time: approx. 30 min + chilling time

Take a ziploc bag and add chicken, lemon juice, garlic and oil to it. Close the bag and keep stirring for 2 minutes until all the ingredients are mixed. Refrigerate for one hour. Heat the grill to medium heat and cook the chicken for 2 minutes on each side. Take a small bowl and mix all the dressing ingredients in it. Place the salad leaves and Parmesan on a serving plate. Drizzle over dressing and mix for good coating. Top with your chicken and parmesan and serve.

Per serving: Cal 529; Net Carbs 5g; Fat 32g; Protein 34g

17.Kale & Broccoli Slaw with Bacon & Parmesan

Ingredients for 2 servings

2 tbsp olive oil
1 cup broccoli slaw
1 cup kale slaw
2 slices bacon, chopped
2 tbsp Parmesan, grated
1 tsp celery seeds
1 ½ tbsp apple cider vinegar
Salt and black pepper to taste

Directions and Total Time: approx. 10 minutes

Take a pan and cook your bacon on medium heat for 5 minutes until crisp. Set the bacon aside to cool. To prepare the salad, take a bowl and mix olive oil, vinegar, salt and pepper in it. Add broccoli, celery seeds and black seeds. Mix well. Serve sprinkled with Parmesan and bacon.

Per serving: Cal 305; Net Carbs 3.7g; Fat 29g; Protein 7g

18.Turkey Bacon & Turnip Salad

Ingredients for 4 servings

2 turnips, cut into wedges
2 tsp olive oil
1/3 cup black olives, sliced
1 cup baby spinach
6 radishes, sliced
3 oz turkey bacon, sliced
4 tbsp buttermilk
2 tsp mustard seeds

1 tsp Dijon mustard
1 tbsp red wine vinegar
Salt and black pepper to taste
1 tbsp chives, chopped

Directions and Total Time: approx. 40 minutes

Take a pan and fry the turkey bacon in it on medium heat until crisp. Take it aside and cut it into pieces. Place baking sheet on parchment paper. Sprinkle olive oil and pepper over it. and bake at 390 F for 30 minutes. Place the baby spinach in the base of the salad plate. And cover with radishes, bacon and turnips. Mix salt, mustard, vinegar and buttermilk. Drizzle the dressing over the salad and toss well then sprinkle with the chives and olives. Serve.

Per serving: Cal 135; Net Carbs 6g; Fat 10g; Protein 6g

19. Chicken, Avocado & Egg Bowls

Ingredients for 2 servings

1 chicken breast, cubed
1 tbsp avocado oil
2 eggs
2 cups green beans
1 avocado, sliced
2 tbsp olive oil
2 tbsp lemon juice
1 tsp Dijon mustard
1 tbsp mint, chopped
Salt and black pepper to taste

Directions and Total Time: approx. 25 minutes

Take a pot and blanch the beans in salted water for 5 minutes until crisp. Rinse off with cold water. Boil eggs in the same hot water for 10 minutes. Remove in an ice bath. Take a pan and heat avocado oil on medium heat. Cook the chicken in the pan for 5 minutes. Remove green beans to two separate salad bowls. Add chicken, egg, avocado slice. Take another bowl and whisk together olive oil, pepper, salt, mustard and lemon juice. Sprinkle over salad. and serve.

Per serving: Cal 692; Net Carbs 6.9g; Fat 53g; Protein 40g

20. Spinach Salad with Pancetta & Mustard

Ingredients for 2 servings

1 cup spinach

1 large avocado, sliced
1 spring onion, sliced
2 pancetta slices
½ lettuce head, shredded
1 hard-boiled egg, chopped Vinaigrette
Salt to taste
¼ tsp garlic powder
3 tbsp olive oil
1 tsp Dijon mustard
1 tbsp white wine vinegar

Directions and Total Time: approx. 20 minutes

Take a pan and fry pancetta slices on medium heat for 5 minutes. Set pancetta aside and let cool. Take a bowl and mix egg, spring onion, spinach, lettuce well. Whisk vinaigrette ingredients in a separate bowl. Pour over the dressing and mix well. Serve immediately with pancetta and avocado.

Per serving: Cal 467; Net Carbs 7g; Fat 42g; Protein 12g

21. Modern Greek Salad with Avocado

Ingredients for 2 servings

1 red bell pepper, roasted and sliced
2 tomatoes, sliced
1 avocado, sliced
6 kalamata olives
¼ lb feta cheese, sliced
1 tbsp vinegar
1 tbsp olive oil
1 tbsp parsley, chopped

Directions and Total Time: approx. 10 minutes

Place the tomatoes on a serving plate. Place avocado slices on it. Top with bell peppers and olives. Place the feta pieces on a plate. Drizzle with vinegar, egg and olive oil. Serve.

Per serving: Cal 411; Net Carbs 5.2g; Fat 35g; Protein 13g

22. Cheesy Beef Salad

Ingredients for 4 servings

½ lb beef rump steak, cut into strips
1 tsp cumin

3 tbsp olive oil
Salt and black pepper to taste
1 tbsp thyme
1 garlic clove, minced
½ cup ricotta, crumbled
½ cup pecans, toasted
2 cups baby spinach
1 ½ tbsp lemon juice
¼ cup fresh mint, chopped

Directions and Total Time: approx. 15 minutes

Heat the grill to medium temperature. Rub the beef with 1 tablespoon olive oil, salt, garlic, black pepper, cumin and thyme. Place on the barbecue and grill for 10 minutes. Take a pan sprinkle pecans and cook for 2 minutes stirring frequently. Cut the grilled beef into strips. Take a bowl and add mint, baby spinach, remaining olive oil, some ricotta, lemon juice, salt and pecans for the salad. Toss thoroughly and add the beef pieces. and serve.

Per serving: Cal 437; Net Carbs 4.2g; Fat 42g; Protein 16g

23.Chicken Salad with Gorgonzola Cheese

Ingredients for 2 servings

½ cup gorgonzola cheese, crumbled
1 chicken breast, boneless, skinless, flattened
Salt and black pepper to taste
1 tbsp garlic powder
2 tsp olive oil
1 cup arugula
1 tbsp red wine vinegar

Directions and Total Time: approx. 15 minutes

Sprinkle garlic powder, salt and black pepper over the meat. Take a pan and heat it on medium heat with half of olive oil. Fry the chicken for 5 minutes until browned on both sides. Let the chicken cool completely. Mix arugula with vinegar and olive oil. Divide the salad and serve with chicken slices on top.

Per serving: Cal 421; Net Carbs 3.5g; Fat 28g; Protein 39g

24. Cheddar & Turkey Meatball Salad

Ingredients for 4 servings

3 tbsp olive oil
1 tbsp lemon juice
1 lb ground turkey
Salt and black pepper to taste
1 head romaine lettuce, torn
2 tomatoes, sliced
¼ red onion, sliced
3 oz yellow cheddar, shredded

Directions and Total Time: approx. 30 minutes

Combine ground turkey with salt and black pepper and form into meatballs. Take a pan and heat half the olive oil in it on medium heat. Fry the meatballs until brown on both sides. Take a salad bowl and mix lettuce, tomatoes and red onions in it. Add olive oil, lemon juice, salt and pepper and mix. Place the meatballs on top. Sprinkle cheese over the salad and serve.

Per serving: Cal 382; Net Carbs 3.5g; Fat 27g; Protein 30g

25. Shrimp Salad with Avocado

Ingredients for 4 servings

2 tomatoes, chopped
½ lb medium shrimp
3 tbsp olive oil
1 avocado, chopped
1 tbsp cilantro, chopped
1 lime, zested and juiced
1 head Iceberg lettuce, torn
Salt and black pepper to taste

Directions and Total Time: approx. 20 minutes

Take a pan and heat 1 tbsp of olive oil on medium heat. And cook the prawns in it for 10 minutes. Take a plate and place salad in it and add tomato, shrimp and avocado. Take another bowl and mix lemon juice, salt, olive oil, pepper in an ice bowl. Garnish with cilantro and serve the salad.

Per serving: Cal 249; Net Carbs 7.2g; Fat 18g; Protein 10g

26. Green Salad with Feta & Blueberries

Ingredients for 4 servings

2 cups broccoli slaw

2 cups baby spinach
2 tbsp poppy seeds
1/3 cup sunflower seeds
1/3 cup blueberries
2/3 cup chopped feta cheese
1/3 cup chopped walnuts
2 tbsp olive oil
1 tbsp white wine vinegar
Salt and black pepper to taste

Directions and Total Time: approx. 10 minutes

Take a bowl and whisk together the poppy seeds, olive oil, vinegar, salt and pepper. And keep it aside. In another bowl, combine the spinach, broccoli slaw, sunflower seeds, walnuts, blueberries and feta cheese. Mix all the ingredients together with the dressing and serve.

Per serving: Cal 301; Net Carbs 7.5g; Fat 24g; Protein 9g

27. Easy Beef Stroganoff

(Ready in about 1 hour | Servings 4)

Ingredients
1 pound beef stew meat, cut across grain into strips
1 cup tomato sauce with garlic and onion
4 ounces fresh mushrooms, sliced
1/2 cup sour cream
2 celery stalks, chopped

Directions

Take a pot and melt 2 teaspoons of lard in it on medium temperature. Roast the meat on all sides for 5 minutes. After that cook until the celery is tender. Add mushrooms and cook for another 5 minutes. Add garlic and onion to the tomato sauce and reduce the heat. Continue cooking for 50 minutes. Remove from heat and serve with sour cream.

Per serving: 303 Calories; 17.2g Fat; 5.6g Carbs 32.4g Protein; 0.9g Fiber

28.Beef Teriyaki with Chinese Cabbage

(Ready in about 15 minutes | Servings 2)

Ingredients

3/4 pound flank steak, thinly sliced

1 yellow onion, thinly sliced
1/2 cup keto teriyaki sauce
1 teaspoon sesame oil
1/2 cup Chinese cabbage, shredded

Directions

Take a pan and heat sesame oil in it on medium temperature. sear the steak and onion for 5 minutes. Add Chinese cabbage and cook for another 5 minutes. Add to Keto Teriyaki Sauce and bring to a boil. Serve immediately when the sauce thickens.

Per serving: 304 Calories; 13.7g Fat; 5.2g Carbs; 37.2g Protein; 0.8g Fiber

29. Chorizo & Tomato Salad with Olives

Ingredients for 4 servings

2 tbsp olive oil
4 chorizo sausages, chopped
2 ½ cups cherry tomatoes
2 tsp red wine vinegar
1 small red onion, chopped
 2 tbsp chopped cilantro
8 sliced Kalamata olives
1 head Boston lettuce, shredded
Salt and black pepper to taste

Directions and Total Time: approx. 10 minutes

Take a large pan and heat 1 tbsp of olive oil in it. Fry the chorizo until golden. Take a bowl and mix vinegar, olive oil, salt and pepper in it. Toss in the onions, tomatoes, lettuce, cilantro and chorizo. Serve with olives.

Per serving: Cal 211; Net Carbs 5.2g; Fat 17g; Protein 10g

30. Beef Stuffed Peppers

(Ready in about 45 minutes | Servings 2)

Ingredients

1/2 pound ground beef
2 bell peppers, deveined and halved
2 tomatoes, pureed
1 garlic clove, minced
Sea salt and ground black pepper, to taste

Directions

Heat a saucepan and brown the ground beef for 5 minutes. Separate with a spatula. Saute the chopped garlic for a minute and sprinkle with salt and ground pepper. Spoon in the chili. Place the peppers in a lightly greased baking dish. Add 1/4 cup water and pureed tomatoes. Bake in preheated oven at 365 F for 40 minutes. and serve.

Per serving: 260 Calories; 14.6g Fat; 6.4g Carbs; 24.2g Protein; 2.2g Fiber

Dinner

1.CRISPY THIGHS & MASH

SERVES 6
PREP TIME: 15 minutes
COOK TIME: 30 minutes

CRISPY CHICKEN:
6 small or 3 large boneless, skinless chicken thighs (about 1 lb/455 g)
¼ cup (60 ml) melted coconut oil or avocado oil
1 teaspoon garlic powder
½ teaspoon onion powder
¼ teaspoon finely ground sea salt
¼ teaspoon ground black pepper

BUTTERNUT MASH:
1 medium butternut squash (about 1¼ lbs/570 g)
2 tablespoons coconut oil or ghee
½ teaspoon finely ground sea salt
⅛ teaspoon ground black pepper
⅓ cup (80 ml) milk (nondairy or regular)
1½ tablespoons chicken bone broth

Cook the Chicken - Preheat the oven to 400 F. Cut the large chicken leg in half. Place the chicken on a rimmed baking sheet. Apply oil on the thigh with spices. Bake for 30 minutes. Cut the chicken into 1/2 inch pieces.

Meanwhile make the mash - peel the squash and remove the seeds. Cut the flesh into cubes. Measure out 3 cup cubes for mash. Keep the remaining squash in the fridge.

Heat oil in a large pan. Add squash, pepper and salt to it. Cover the pan and cook the squash for 15 minutes. Add mutton broth and milk to it and cover and cook again for 15 minutes. Once the squash is done, mash with the back of a fork. Add an equal amount of thighs to the chicken and serve.

Per serving, made with coconut oil and full-fat coconut milk:

calories: 331 | calories from fat: 239 | total fat: 26.5 g | saturated fat: 13.1 g | cholesterol: 91 mg sodium: 613 mg | carbs: 9.9 g | dietary fiber: 1.6 g | net carbs: 8.3 g | sugars: 1.8 g | protein: 16.2 g FAT: 70% CARBS: 11% PROTEIN: 19%

2.NOODLES & GLAZED SALMON

SERVES 4
PREP TIME : 5 minutes
COOK TIME : 20 minutes

1/4 cup plus 2 tablespoons (75 ml) avocado oil, divided
¼ cup (60 ml) coconut aminos
2 tablespoons plus 2 teaspoons tomato paste
2 tablespoons apple cider vinegar
1 (2-in/5-cm) piece fresh ginger root, grated
4 cloves garlic, minced
½ teaspoon finely ground sea salt
1 pound (455 g) salmon fillets, cut into 4 equal portions
2 (7-oz/198-g) packages konjac noodles or equivalent amount of other low-carb noodles of choice
2 green onions, sliced
Handful of fresh cilantro leaves, roughly chopped
1 teaspoon sesame seeds

Take a large pan and heat oil in it. Let the oil get heated and make the sauce. Take a small bowl and mix together tomato paste, vinegar, ginger, garlic, salt, coconut aminos, remaining 1/4 cup of oil. Lower the heat of the hot pan and place the salmon in it. Slather with sauce. Add the rest of the sauce to the pan. Cover and cook on medium heat for 15-20 minutes. Once the salmon is done, move it to one side of the pan to make room for the noodles. Add noodles and green onions to the pan. Mix well to coat with remaining sauce. Place the cooked salmon on top of the noodles. Cook for another 4 minutes to heat the noodles a little more. Sprinkle the sesame seeds and cilantro on top of the salmon. Serve with pan sauce.

Per serving, made with konjac noodles:

calories: 333 | calories from fat: 202 | total fat: 22.4 g | saturated fat: 2.5 g | cholesterol: 45 mg sodium: 287 mg | carbs: 8.2 g | dietary fiber: 3.6 g | net carbs: 4.6 g | sugars: 0.9 g | protein: 24.7 g FAT :61% CARBS: 10% PROTEIN: 30%

3.SCALLOPS & MOZZA BROCCOLI MASH

SERVES 4
PREP TIME: 5 minutes
COOK TIME: 35 minutes

MOZZA BROCCOLI MASH:

¼ cup (55 g) coconut oil or ghee, or ¼ cup (60 ml) avocado oil
6 cups (570 g) broccoli florets
4 cloves garlic, minced
1 (2-in/5-cm) piece fresh ginger root, grated
⅔ cup (160 ml) chicken bone broth
½ cup (70 g) shredded mozzarella cheese (dairy-free or regular)

SCALLOPS:
1 pound (455 g) sea scallops
¼ teaspoon finely ground sea salt
¼ teaspoon ground black pepper
2 tablespoons coconut oil, avocado oil, or ghee
Lemon wedges, for serving

Prepare the mash first. Heat oil in a pan on medium temperature. Add ginger, garlic and broccoli and cook for 5 minutes. Add the mutton stock and cover. Cook on medium heat for 30 minutes. Prepare the scallops 5 minutes before the broccoli is ready. Pat the scallops dry and add pepper and salt on both sides. Heat oil in a small pan on medium heat. When the oil is hot, add the scallops. Cook on each side. When the broccoli is done, add the cheese and mash it with a fork. Serve with lemon wedges.

Per serving, made with coconut oil and dairy-free cheese:

calories: 353 | calories from fat: 229 | total fat: 25.4 g | saturated fat: 19.9 g | cholesterol: 27 mg sodium: 768 mg | carbs: 12 g | dietary fiber: 7 g | net carbs: 5 g | sugars: 1 g | protein: 19.2 g FAT: 65% CARBS: 14% PROTEIN: 22%

4.BBQ BEEF & SLAW

SERVES 4
PREP TIME: 10 minutes
COOK TIME: 45 minutes or 4 to 6 hours, depending on method

BBQ BEEF:
1 pound (455 g) boneless beef chuck roast
1 cup (240 ml) beef bone broth
½ teaspoon finely ground sea salt
½ cup (80 g) sugar-free barbecue sauce

SLAW:
9 ounces (255 g) coleslaw mix
½ cup (120 ml) sugar-free poppy seed dressing

Put the salt, stock and chuck roast in a pressure cooker. Close the lid of the pressure cooker and cook on high pressure for 50 minutes. Naturally release the pressure after completion. Cook for at least 4 hours or 6 hours if you are using a slow cooker. Once the meat is done, drain it completely, leaving 1/4 cup of the cooking liquid in the cooker. Shred the meat with two forks, add the barbecue sauce and mix to coat. Place the coleslaw mix and dressing in a salad bowl. Toss to coat. Serve and enjoy.

Per serving, made with Quick 'n' Easy Barbecue Sauce and homemade poppy seed dressing:

calories: 354 | calories from fat: 240 | total fat: 26.7 g | saturated fat: 4.7 g | cholesterol: 70 mg sodium: 566 mg | carbs: 4.6 g | dietary fiber: 1.7 g | net carbs: 2.9 g | sugars: 2.5 g | protein: 23.9 g FAT: 68% CARBS: 5% PROTEIN: 27%

5.CREAM OF MUSHROOM–STUFFED CHICKEN

SERVES 4
PREP TIME: 10 minutes
COOK TIME: 45 minutes

3 tablespoons coconut oil, avocado oil, or ghee
7 ounces (200 g) cremini mushrooms, chopped
4 cloves garlic, minced
3 teaspoons dried parsley, divided
¾ teaspoon finely ground sea salt, divided
¼ teaspoon ground black pepper
1 pound (455 g) boneless, skin-on chicken breasts
1 teaspoon onion powder
1 teaspoon garlic powder
½ cup (120 ml) milk (nondairy or regular)
4 cups (280 g) spinach, for serving

Preheat oven to 400 F. Line a baking sheet lined with parchment paper. Heat oil in a large pan over medium heat. Add garlic, 2 teaspoons of eggs, mushrooms, 1/4 teaspoon of salt and pepper and saute for 10 minutes. Using a knife, tear the belly of the chicken breast into 2 parts. Place the chicken breasts on a baking sheet. Place 1/4 of the mushroom mixture in the center of each open breast. Fold the breast over to cover the filling. Pour the milk directly into the pan between the chicken breasts. Bake the chicken for 30 minutes. Drizzle the spinach with the creamy pan juices. and serve.

Per serving, made with coconut oil and full-fat coconut milk:

calories: 388 | calories from fat: 219 | total fat: 24.3 g | saturated fat: 11.4 g | cholesterol: 96 mg sodium: 492 mg | carbs: 6.6 g | dietary fiber: 2.3 g | net carbs: 4.3 g | sugars: 1.6 g | protein: 38.2 g FAT: 55% CARBS: 7% PROTEIN: 38%

6.PORK CHOPS

SERVES 4

INGREDIENTS
½ tsp. peppercorns

1 medium star anise
1 stalk lemongrass
4 halved garlic cloves
4 pork chops (boneless)
1 tbsp. fish sauce
1 tbsp. almond flour
1½ tsp. soy sauce
1 tsp. sesame oil
½ tsp. five spice
½ tbsp. sambal chili paste
½ tbsp. sugar free ketchup

DIRECTIONS

Take a blender and grind the pepper and star anise. Take a food processor and add the soy sauce, fish sauce, sesame oil, five spice, garlic, pepper powder and star anise and blend until combined. Place the pork on a tray and marinate for 2 hours. Cover the pork slices with almond flour. Make sure that the dohi is seared on both sides by frying on high temperature. Remove and cut into strips. Serve.

NUTRITIONAL INFO PER SERVING

Calories: 224 Fat: 10g Net Carbs: 5g Protein: 35g

7. PORK HOCK

SERVES 2

INGREDIENTS
1 lb. pork hock
¼ cup rice vinegar
⅓ cup soy sauce
⅓ cup shaoxing cooking wine
¼ cup sweetener
⅓ onion
1 tbsp. butter
Shiitake mushrooms
1 tsp. Chinese five-spice
1 tsp. oregano
2 crushed garlic cloves

DIRECTIONS

Take a pan and fry onions in it. Meanwhile, boil the mushrooms until they are tender. Take another pan and fry the pork in it. After a while, add all the ingredients to the Crock-Pot and cook on high for 2 hours, then stir and cook for another 2 hours. Remove the pork and slice it back into the pot to absorb more flavor. Serve with vegetables.

NUTRITIONAL INFO PER SERVING

Calories: 550 Fat: 32g Net Carbs: 20g Protein: 50g

8.MEATBALLS WITH BACON AND CHEESE

SERVES 5

INGREDIENTS
1½ lb. ground beef
¾ cup pork rinds, crushed
¾ tsp. salt
¾ tsp. pepper
¾ tsp. cumin
¾ tsp. garlic powder
¾ cup cheddar cheese
4 slices bacon
1 egg

DIRECTIONS

First process the pork rinds to form a powder. Add garlic powder, ground beef, salt, pork, pepper, cumin and cheese and mix well. Cut the bacon into small pieces and fry in a hot pan. After cooling, add the bacon and mix well. Prepare the meatballs. Cook the meatballs in a pan. Cover for 10 minutes and serve with your choice of sauce.

NUTRITIONAL INFO PER SERVING
Calories: 450 Fat: 26g Net Carbs: 3g Protein: 50g

9.BACON WRAPPED CHICKEN

SERVES 4

INGREDIENTS
2 skinless chicken breasts, boneless
2 oz. blue cheese
4 slices ham
8 slices bacon

DIRECTIONS

Tear the belly of the breast and cut it in half. Place 2 slices of ham and cheese in the center. Cover the entire breast and wrap with 4 slices of bacon. Place the breasts in an ovenproof skillet. Remove from pan and cook in oven at 325 F. Allow to cool and serve after 10 minutes.

NUTRITIONAL INFO PER SERVING

Calories: 270 Fat: 11g Net Carbs: 0.50g Protein: 38g

10. SAUSAGE & CABBAGE SKILLET MELT

SERVES 4

INGREDIENTS
4 spicy Italian chicken sausages
1½ cups green cabbage, shredded
1½ cups purple cabbage, shredded
½ cup onion, diced
2 tsp. coconut oil
2 slices Colby jack cheese
2 tsp. fresh cilantro, chopped

DIRECTIONS

First fry onion and cabbage. Take a kadai, melt coconut oil in it and fry cabbage and onion on medium temperature and cook for 10 minutes. Add the sausage and let it mix with the vegetables and cook for another 10 minutes. Add cheese on top. Cover and switch off the gas. Serve after cooling.

NUTRITIONAL INFO PER SERVING

Calories: 233 Fat: 15g Net Carbs: 5g Protein: 20g

11.SPAGHETTI SQUASH WITH MEAT SAUCE

SERVES 8

INGREDIENTS
2 spaghetti squashes
2 lb. ground beef
33-oz. jar of spaghetti sauce
1 tbsp. minced garlic
1 tbsp. Italian seasoning
Parmesan cheese

DIRECTIONS

Cut the spaghetti squash in half and scoop out the guts. Take a glass container half filled with water and cook the remaining crust and meat at 375 F for 50 minutes until tender. Fry the beef on the stove at medium temperature and mix with spices, sauces. Remove spaghetti and serve with sauce.

NUTRITIONAL INFO PER SERVING

Calories: 170 Fat: 15g Net Carbs: 12g Protein: 11g

12.CHEESY BACON BRUSSELS SPROUTS

SERVES 4

INGREDIENTS
5 slices bacon
16 oz. Brussels sprouts
6 oz. cheddar cheese

DIRECTIONS

Cut the bacon into small pieces and fry until crisp. Chop the Brussels sprouts in a food processor. Fry bacon in grease until tender. When the Brussels sprouts are crisp, add the bacon and cheese. Cook until the cheese melts. Serve.

NUTRITIONAL INFO PER SERVING

Calories: 260 Fat: 22g Net Carbs: 5g Protein: 17g

13. PARMESAN CHICKEN

SERVES 4

INGREDIENTS
For the Chicken:
3 chicken breasts
1 cup mozzarella cheese
Salt and pepper
For the Coating:
2½ oz. pork rinds
¼ cup flaxseed meal
½ cup parmesan cheese
1 tsp. oregano
½ tsp. salt
½ tsp. pepper
¼ tsp. red pepper flakes
½ tsp. garlic
2 tsp. paprika
1 egg
1½ tsp. chicken broth

The Sauce
¼ cup olive oil
1 cup tomato sauce
½ tsp. garlic
½ tsp. oregano
Salt and pepper

DIRECTIONS

Take a food processor and grind the parmesan cheese, spices and pork rinds. Cut the chicken breasts into three pieces. Season them with pepper and salt. Take another bowl and make a coating by beating eggs and adding chicken broth. Start making the sauce by taking a pan and start mixing all the sauce ingredients in it. Let it boil for 20 minutes. Dip the chicken pieces in the egg mixture and dip the pork in the coating. and place on foil. Take a pan and fry chicken with two spoons of olive oil. Place the fried chicken in a casserole dish and bake at 400 F for 10 minutes.

NUTRITIONAL INFO PER SERVING

Calories: 646 Fat: 47g Net Carbs: 5g Protein: 49g

14. CREAMY CHICKEN

SERVES 1

INGREDIENTS
5 oz. chicken breast
1 tbsp. olive oil
3 oz. mushrooms
¼ small onion, sliced
½ cup chicken broth
¼ cup heavy cream
½ tsp. dried tarragon
1 tsp. grain mustard
Salt and pepper

DIRECTIONS

First cut the chicken into cubes and season. Take a pan and fry it in olive oil and take it out on a plate. In the same pan add onion and mushroom and saute. Add chicken broth to it and reduce by boiling for 5 minutes. Add chicken, spices and remaining ingredients and simmer for another 5 minutes. Serve.

NUTRITIONAL INFO PER SERVING

Calories: 489 Fat: 43g Net Carbs: 5g Protein: 30g

15. LOW CARB CHICKEN NUGGETS

SERVES 4

INGREDIENTS
For the Nuggets:
24 oz. chicken thighs
1 egg
For the Crust:
1½ oz. pork rinds
¼ cup flax meal
¼ cup almond meal
Zest of 1 lime
⅛ tsp. garlic powder
¼ tsp. paprika
¼ tsp. chili powder
⅛ tsp. onion powder
⅛ tsp. cayenne pepper
¼ tsp. salt
¼ tsp. pepper
For the Sauce:
½ cup mayonnaise
½ avocado
¼ tsp. garlic powder
1 tbsp. lime juice
⅛ tsp. cumin
½ tsp. red chili flakes

DIRECTIONS

Pat the chicken dry and cut into bite-sized pieces. Take a food processor and mix the crust ingredients in it. Take a bowl and separate the crumbs and the beaten egg. Dip the chicken in the egg, coat and then place on a greased baking sheet. Bake in the oven at 400 F for 20 minutes. Mix all the sauce ingredients together to make the sauce. Serve and be happy.

NUTRITIONAL INFO PER SERVING

Calories: 615 Fat: 53g Net Carbs: 2g Protein: 39g

16. TOTCHOS

SERVES 2

INGREDIENTS
2 servings keto tater tots

6 oz. ground beef
2 oz. shredded cheddar cheese
2 tbsp. sour cream
6 sliced black olives
1 tbsp. salsa
½ jalapeño pepper, sliced

DIRECTIONS

Take a small pan and add 10 tots, half the ground beef and half the cheese. Add some more tots on top. Also add the rest of the meat and cheese. Roast in the oven for 5 minutes and serve with black cream, sour cream, salsa and jalapeño.

NUTRITIONAL INFO PER SERVING
Calories: 638 Fat: 53g Net Carbs: 6g Protein: 32g

17. PORK PIES

SERVES 4

INGREDIENTS
1 lb. ground pork
4 tbsp. grated parmesan cheese
2 beaten eggs
½ tsp. ground nutmeg
½ tsp. ginger
½ tsp. cardamom
½ lemon zest
4 tart shells (keto)
Salt and pepper

DIRECTIONS

Take a pan and put meat and spices in it. When it cooks a little, add the egg and lemon. Spoon some of the mixture into keto pie shells and bake for 30 minutes. Remove from oven and serve when cool.

NUTRITIONAL INFO PER SERVING

Calories: 560 Fat: 23g Net Carbs: 6g Protein: 30g

18. GLAZED SALMON

SERVES 2

INGREDIENTS

10 oz. salmon filet
2 tbsp. soy sauce
2 tsp. sesame oil
1 tbsp. rice vinegar
1 tsp. ginger, minced
2 tsp. garlic minced
1 tbsp. red boat fish sauce
1 tbsp. sugar free ketchup
2 tbsp. white wine

DIRECTIONS

Add remaining ingredients except ketchup, sesame oil, white wine in a container and marinate the salmon for 15 minutes. Heat sesame oil in a pan on high heat. Place the file skin side down. Cook until both sides are crispy and remove the fish to prepare the glaze. Add the white wine and ketchup to the marinade. Place in pan and simmer for 5 minutes.

NUTRITIONAL INFO PER SERVING

Calories: 372 Fat: 24g Net Carbs: 3g Protein: 35g

19. COCONUT SHRIMP

SERVES 3

INGREDIENTS
For the Coconut Shrimp:
1 lb. peeled and de-veined shrimp
2 egg whites
1 cup unsweetened coconut flakes
2 tbsp. coconut flour
For the Sweet Chili Dipping Sauce:
½ cup sugar free apricot preserves
1 ½ tsp. rice wine vinegar
1 tbsp. lime juice
1 medium diced red chili
¼ tsp. red pepper flakes

DIRECTIONS

Beat the egg white until soft. Take two separate bowls and put coconut flour and coconut flakes in them. Dip the prawns, egg whites then coconut pieces in the coconut batter. Place shrimp on a baking sheet and bake at 400 F for 15 minutes. Also fry for 5 minutes until crisp. Mix all the ingredients to make a sauce and serve with the sauce.

NUTRITIONAL INFO PER SERVING

Calories: 398 Fat: 22g Net Carbs: 7g Protein: 36g

20.Cheesy Eggplant Casserole

Serves: 2
Time: 35 Minutes

Ingredients:
2 Eggplants
2 Tablespoons Olive Oil
1 ½ Cups Mozzarella Cheese, Grated
1 ½ Cups Marinara Sauce
½ Cup Parmesan Cheese
Sea Salt to Taste
1 Tomato, Sliced
Basil, Fresh & Chopped to Garnish
Sea Salt & Black Pepper to Taste

Directions:

Preheat the oven to 350 F. Line a baking tray with aluminum foil. Grease with a spoon of olive oil. Cut eggplant into thin slices and sprinkle salt on it. Place on a baking tray. Bake for 3 minutes and cook for 3 minutes. Take out the oven tray and set the pieces aside without turning off the oven. Take a casserole dish and grease it with 1 tbsp of olive oil. Add 1/3 of the marinara sauce and Parmesan cheese. Place a layer of eggplants first and then add the mozzarella.
Repeat this process until all the ingredients are combined in your dish, except for some parmesan. Top with a final layer of tomatoes and parmesan cheese. Sprinkle with black pepper. Bake in the oven for 20 minutes or until the cheese is browned. Serve chilled. Preheat the oven to 350 F. Line a baking tray with aluminum foil. Grease with a spoon of olive oil. Cut eggplant into thin slices and sprinkle salt on it. Place on a baking tray. Bake for 3 minutes and cook for 3 minutes. Take out the oven tray and set the pieces aside without turning off the oven.

Take a casserole dish and grease it with 1 tbsp of olive oil. Add 1/3 of the marinara sauce and Parmesan cheese. Place a layer of eggplants first and then add the mozzarella. Repeat this process until all the ingredients are combined in your dish, except for some parmesan. Top with a final layer of tomatoes and parmesan cheese. Sprinkle with black pepper. Bake in the oven for 20 minutes or until the cheese is browned. Serve chilled.

Calories: 496 Protein: 28 Grams Fat: 39 Grams Net Carbs: 8.1 Grams

21. Spinach & Mushroom Casserole

Serves: 6
Time: 1 Hour 30 Minutes

Calories: 149
Protein: 8.5 Grams
Fat: 9.4 Grams
Net Carbs: 3.9 Grams

Ingredients:
1 Celery Root, Large & Cubed
8 Ounces Baby Portobello Mushrooms, Quartered
1 Cup Vegetable Broth
3 Eggs
2 Cloves Garlic, Minced
2 Tablespoons Olive Oil
1 Onion, Diced
10 Ounces Spinach
1 ½ Cups Coconut Milk
½ Teaspoon Nutmeg
Parsley, Fresh & Chopped Fine to Garnish
Sea Salt & Black Pepper to Taste

Directions:

Preheat the oven to 350 F. To make the rice, chop the celery in a food processor. Heat a pan and oil on medium heat. Cook onion in it for 3 minutes. Also add garlic and let it cook for a minute. Add mushrooms and cook for another 5 minutes. Add spinach and cook for another 5 minutes. Take a bowl and beat nutmeg, milk, broth, eggs in it. Take out the baking dish. Add to your egg mixture and bake for 50 minutes. Serve.

22. Beef & Spinach Casserole

Serves: 4
Time: 55 Minutes
Calories: 484
Protein: 35 Grams
Fat: 36 Grams
Net Carbs: 1.5 Grams

Ingredients:
1 lb. Ground Beef
Sea Salt & Black Pepper to Taste
1 Tomato, Sliced
2 Cups Baby Spinach
1 Cup Black Olives, Sliced
1 Tablespoon Cilantro, Fresh
8 Egg
½ Cup Parmesan Cheese, Grated

Directions:

...ry in a food processor. Heat a pan and oil on ...and let it cook for a minute. Add mushrooms ...er 5 minutes. Take a bowl and beat nutmeg, ...mixture and bake for 50 minutes. Serve.

...& Canned
...soning
...heese

...ons:

Heat the slow cooker to medium heat. Take out a medium pan. Heat the ground beef on medium heat. Fry the meat for 10 minutes. Sprinkle salt and pepper over it. Take a slow cooker and cook tomatoes, ground beef, taco seasoning, beef broth and cream cheese on low for 4 hours. Stir occasionally to prevent burning. Ladle five bowls. and serve.

24. Bacon & Zucchini Casserole

Serves: 5
Time: 40 Minutes
Calories: 496
Protein: 19 Grams
Fat: 48 Grams
Net Carbs: 3.5 Grams

Ingredients:
1 Tablespoon Lard
1 lb. Bacon, Sliced into Strips
1 Spring Onion, Diced Fine
3 Zucchinis, Large
Sea Salt & Black Pepper to Taste
6 Eggs

70

½ Container Feta Cheese, Crumbled

Directions:

Preheat the oven to 350 F. Then take out the casserole dish. Grease the casserole dish with lard. And then put the bacon on the bottom. Then top with green onions and sliced zucchini rings. Sprinkle with pepper and salt. Take a bowl and beat eggs in it then add salt and feta cheese. Mix well and add to casserole dish. Cook for half an hour and serve hot.

25.Chicken & Artichoke Casserole

Serves: 4
Time: 35 Minutes
Calories: 101
Protein: 22 Grams
Fat: 29 Grams
Net Carbs: 2.5 Grams

Ingredients:
2 Tablespoons Butte
11 Ounces Artichoke Hearts, Drained
2 Green Onions, Chopped
1 Chicken Breast, Cubed
½ Cup White Wine, dry
1 Tablespoon Almond Flour
½ Cup Bone Broth
½ Cup Cream
¼ Teaspoon Tarragon Leaves
2 Tablespoons Parsley, Chopped for Garnish
Sea Salt & Black Pepper to Taste

Directions:

Preheat the oven to 350 F. Then take out the casserole dish and grease it with butter. Cut the artichokes and place them in the bottom of the casserole dish. Add green onions and chicken cubes to it. Take a bowl and mix it well with almond flour, bone broth, wine and cream. Your almond flour should dissolve completely. After that take out this mixture in a casserole dish. Cook for 20 minutes and serve hot.

26.Chicken Curry Casserole

Serves: 4
Time: 35 Minutes
Calories: 186
Protein: 26 Grams
Fat: 8 Grams
Net Carbs: 4 Grams

Ingredients:
1 lb. Chicken Breast, Cubed
1 Tablespoon Chicken Fat
1 Onion, Sliced Fine
1 Carrot
2 Teaspoons Curry Powder
1 Pinch Saffron
½ Cup Wine
½ Cup Bone Broth
1 Tablespoon Coriander, Fresh
Sea Salt to Taste

Directions:

Cut the chicken breasts into cubes. Then take a pan and heat the chicken fat in it, return the onion to medium heat. Add your chicken cubes to the pan and cook until browned. Stir well and sprinkle saffron and curry. Stir well and add bone broth and wine. Stir well and sprinkle with salt. Cover and let it simmer for 25 minutes. Sprinkle coriander and serve.

27. Asparagus Stuffed Chicken Breasts

Serves: 4
Time: 45 Minutes
Calories: 236
Protein: 32 Grams
Fat: 30 Grams
Net Carbs: 1.8 Grams

Ingredients:
2 Chicken Breasts Halves, Skinless & Boneless
8 Asparagus Spears, Trimmed
½ Cup Parmesan Cheese, Shredded
¼ Cup Ground Almonds
Sea Salt & Black Pepper to Taste

Directions:

Preheat the oven to 375 F. Then grease the baking dish. Keep the baking dish aside. Place each chicken breast between freezer bags and flatten slightly before placing on a flat surface before sprinkling with salt and pepper. Place four spears in the center of each and then top with 1/4 cup Parmesan. Repeat the same process with the remaining chicken breasts and then roll them well. Place the rolls in a baking dish. Sprinkle two tablespoons of ground almonds over each chicken breast. Bake for 30 minutes and serve when cool.

28. Celery & Grouper Casserole

Serves: 8
Time: 25 Minutes
Calories: 371
Protein: 23 Grams
Fat: 29 Grams
Net Carbs: 1.9 Grams

Ingredients:
3 ½ lbs. Grouper Fish
1 ½ lbs. Celery, Fresh & Chopped
1 Cup Olive Oil
½ Cup White Wine
Sea Salt & Black Pepper to Taste
1 Lemon, Juiced

Directions:

Season the grouper with salt and pepper. Then wash the celery and place it in a large saucepan. Place the fish pieces on top of the celery and add the lemon juice, olive oil and vinegar to the pan. Cook on high until boiling. Cook on medium heat for 5 minutes. Season with salt and pepper and serve hot.

29.Shrimp & Broccoli

Serves: 4
Time: 30 Minutes
Calories: 220
Protein: 27 Grams
Fat: 10 Grams
Net Carbs: 6.3 Grams

Ingredients:
2 Tablespoons Sesame Oil
4 Cloves Garlic, Minced
1 Cup Water
2 Teaspoons Ginger Root, Fresh & Grated
2 Tablespoons Coconut Aminos
2 Cups Broccoli Florets, Fresh
1 ½ lbs. Shrimp, Peeled & Deveined
Lemon Wedges for Garnish

Directions:

Heat a large pan over medium heat and add the garlic. Let the garlic cook for 5 minutes. Add water, coconut aminos and ginger. Bring this mixture to a boil. Cook the prawns for 5 minutes. Add the broccoli and cook for another 10 minutes. Serve hot with lemon wedges before garnishing.

30.Broccoli & Bacon Casserole

Serves: 4
Time: 50 Minutes
Calories: 325
Protein: 22 Grams
Fat: 24 Grams
Net Carbs: 4.8 Grams

Ingredients:
1 Tablespoon Olive oil
2 Cups Broccoli Florets, Cooked
8 Eggs
¼ Cup Water
1 Cup Cottage Cheese
1 Teaspoon Thyme, fresh & Chopped
Sea Salt & Black Pepper to Taste
3 Ounces Bacon, Crumbled
2 Tablespoons Feta Cheese, Crumbled

Directions:

Preheat the oven to 380 F. Take out the casserole dish. Coat with olive oil. Place the broccoli on the bottom and sprinkle with pepper and salt. Add thyme and cottage cheese. Take a bowl and beat your eggs with 1/4 of water, pepper and salt. Add egg mixture to it. Beat the crumbs and add the bacon. Cook for 30 minutes. Serve when cooled.

Part 3

Frequently Asked Rarely Answered Questions

How to overcome eating food that is not on diet plan temptation?

Be aware of your thoughts when you feel food cravings. Research has found that taking some time to prepare your mental and physical state to avoid eating the wrong foods can kill cravings. Imagine the reward for making the right decisions e.g. imagine yourself 10 pounds lighter so imagine how you will look and feel if you consistently eat healthy. Research has found that imagining the consequences of bad decisions can help people make better decisions.

Research has shown that when you're tempted to eat the wrong food, tell yourself I'll eat it later. Research shows that often deciding to eat something later is enough to stop the craving, and chances are the craving will go away shortly after. Change your cravings if you are really hungry but instead of eating unhealthy, get yourself into the habit of eating healthy food.

Distract Yourself. When you feel a food craving, try to treat yourself to something else. Boredom or fatigue often leads to cravings for food, but mostly keeping yourself busy will help you stay away from either of these. Getting plenty of sleep. A lack of sleep can make your body need more calories and this is linked to junk food cravings.

Celebrate any festival in moderation. Tasty but unhealthy foods are part of many of our celebrations. Clean Out Your Cupboards. The only way to make sure you don't eat unhealthy foods at home is to keep them out of your home. House Waste Anna Keep Out of Sight R & Keep Healthy Food Available. The flip side of hiding junk food from you is making sure healthier options are more easily seen and accessible, making you more likely to eat them instead.

How to avoid sugar?

Eat a little. Eat what you want in small amounts as dietitians recommend eating a small cookie or candy bar. Eating small amounts of what you like helps to remove negative emotions from the mind. If you want to avoid sugar cravings altogether, try chewing a stick of gum. Research has shown that chewing gum can reduce food cravings. When sugar cravings hit, make it a habit to eat fruit so you get the nutrients in the form of fiber along with the sweetness.

Eat Regular Meals. Waiting too long between meals can predispose you to choosing foods high in fat and high in sugar. Don't be ashamed to seek help. Many people turn to sweets when they're stressed, depressed or angry, but food doesn't solve emotional problems.

How to take critical vitamins?

Vitamins and minerals are very essential for life. They not only keep you healthy but also make you efficient and protect you from various diseases. Vitamins and minerals are mentioned together but are completely different. Vitamins are organic substances produced by plants or animals. They are called essential because they cannot be synthesized in the body, so they must be obtained from the body. Minerals are inorganic elements that originate from water, soil, and rocks.

Following a healthy diet is important to ensure you get a variety of vitamins and minerals. These include fruits, vegetables, whole grains, beans and legumes, low-fat versions, and dairy products. Many common foods contain minerals and vitamins, making it easy to meet your daily needs from food. Here are some of the best foods for vitamins and minerals important for the body, according to the Harvard Medical School Special Health Report.

Vitamin Sources

Water soluble:

B-1: ham, soymilk, watermelon, acorn squash

B-2: milk, yogurt, cheese, whole and enriched grains and cereals.

B-3: meat, poultry, fish, fortified and whole grains, mushrooms, potatoes

B-5: chicken, whole grains, broccoli, avocados, mushrooms

B-6: meat, fish, poultry, legumes, tofu and other soy products, bananas

B-7: Whole grains, eggs, soybeans, fish

B-9: Fortified grains and cereals, asparagus, spinach, broccoli, legumes (black-eyed peas and chickpeas), orange juice

B-12: Meat, poultry, fish, milk, cheese, fortified soymilk and cereals

Vitamin C: Citrus fruit, potatoes, broccoli, bell peppers, spinach, strawberries, tomatoes, Brussels sprouts

Fat soluble:

Vitamin A: beef, liver, eggs, shrimp, fish, fortified milk, sweet potatoes, carrots, pumpkins, spinach, mangoes

Vitamin D: Fortified milk and cereals, fatty fish

Vitamin E: vegetables oils, leafy green vegetables, whole grains, nuts

Vitamin K: Cabbage, eggs, milk, spinach, broccoli, kale

Minerals

Major:

Calcium: yogurt, cheese, milk, salmon, leafy green vegetables

Chloride: salt

Magnesium: Spinach, broccoli, legumes, seeds, whole-wheat bread

Potassium: meat, milk, fruits, vegetables, grains, legumes

Sodium: salt, soy sauce, vegetables

Trace:

Chromium: meat, poultry, fish, nuts, cheese

Copper: shellfish, nuts, seeds, whole-grain products, beans, prunes

Fluoride: fish, teas

Iodine: Iodized salt, seafood

Iron: red meat, poultry, eggs, fruits, green vegetables, fortified bread

Manganese: nuts, legumes, whole grains, tea

Selenium: Organ meat, seafood, walnuts

Zinc: meat, shellfish, legumes, whole grains

What foods can I eat to help keep me full longer?

Fruits, vegetables, and whole grains have high water and fiber content that provide volume and weight but less calories. Changing your unhealthy habits isn't easy, but knowing which foods are good for energy density is the first step.

Many of these vegetables are very low in calories because the vegetables contain water and fiber that provides weight without the calories. To include more vegetables in your diet, reduce meat portions and increase servings of vegetables. Add vegetables to your sandwiches. Eat raw vegetables for breakfast.

Fruit juices are a concentrated source of natural sugars so they tend to be high in calories and don't fill you up as much. On the contrary, eating fresh frozen fruits is a better option. Because they contain less calories than fruit juice and eating fruits makes you feel full for a long time. Whole grains are still the best choice because they contain fiber and other important nutrients. Choose whole grain options instead of refined grains and foods made with sugar or white flour. E.g. Whole-wheat bread, Whole-wheat pasta, Oatmeal, Brown rice, Whole-grain cereal

The healthiest low energy dense options are foods high in protein but low in fat and calories. Beans, peas and lentils, Fish, Lean meat and poultry, Low-fat or fat-free dairy products, such as milk, yogurt and cheese, Egg whites

Although fats are highly energy dense foods, some fats are healthier than others, such as monounsaturated and polyunsaturated fats. Include them in your meals. Such as olive, flaxseed and safflower oils contain healthy fats. Limit the amount of saturated fat and trans fat in your diet.

Our family won't support for our diet

Researchers say it can be very difficult when only one family member is trying to change their eating habits, and other family members either don't need to change or don't really want to. You feel that you should be supported by your family but you are not sure how exactly your family should support you.

We tell our family that you should support me in my diet but we don't tell them clearly how to support. So there is no match between their thoughts and ours. So conflict happens. Eventually we get frustrated and so do our family members. The solution is to take a pen and paper and clearly write down what you need in terms of their support and show it to them. Also tell them how they should support. Instead of saying help me, give them specific ideas about what you would like them to do or not do.

Experts say that it is only in your hands to make a diet plan successful and not dependent on others. It is said that the thoughts of the five people you hang out with every day affect your thoughts and you become like them after a while. That's why it's important to connect with people who are trying to lose weight like you, and Join Facebook Groups for that. Share your daily progress with your friends, also share the problems you face and ask solutions from them.

Keep healthy foods on the shopping list to avoid temptation when going to the supermarket. Ask family members to eat out high-calorie foods. Plan meals for five days a week and let your family members do it for two days.

The greatest challenge is eating out with friends, family on diet

Before going to a restaurant, read the menu and plan what you are going to eat. You won't regret it later by choosing your food before you go. Eat a healthy snack before going to a restaurant. If you're hungry after going to a restaurant, you're more likely to overeat, so eat a healthy breakfast before you go to prevent this. Yogurt is low in calories and high in protein, so it can be a great option for healthy snacks.

Drink a full glass of water before meals to reduce your appetite. One study showed that people who drank 500 ml of water before a meal ate fewer calories and therefore lost 44% more weight. Check how the food is cooked in the restaurant as the way the food is cooked can have a significant effect on the calorie content. Try to stay away from fried foods as they are high in calories. Have a cup of coffee instead of dessert.

Chances are you will overeat in a buffet style meal. A great option to avoid this is to use small dishes for eating. Order soup before you start so you can stop overeating. Studies looking at the effects of eating soup before a meal have shown that it can reduce your total calorie intake by 20 percent.

How to get consistency on a 1200 calorie diet?

Make it a habit to check the calories on everything and choose foods with fewer calories. It may not seem like much that you can easily save 50 calories per container by choosing low-calorie yogurt, but if you can save 50 calories per meal, you'll gain another 150 calories, which is enough for extra consumption.

Count all the calories you eat. I see many people following diet plans who think that counting small food is not important. If you are on a 3000-3500 calorie diet it is not so important. But when you are following a 1200 calorie diet plan then the calories of food like apple are also important as it contains 100 calories.

Focus on protein. When you follow a 1200 calorie diet plan, it is very important to pay attention to the food you eat. Because protein helps you feel fuller for longer. When I was following a 1200 calorie diet plan, eating yogurt made me feel fuller longer than eating bananas, and I was in a better mood throughout the day.

Eat low calorie vegetables in your diet. According to researchers, people around the world are eating more ultra-processed foods than ever before. Ultra processed foods include fast food frozen dinners and sugary sodas. If you manage to keep these foods out of the house, you can help avoid the temptation to eat them by limiting access to them.

Restaurant meals are higher in calories, sugar, fat, and highly processed foods than home-cooked meals, and they tend to be larger in size, so maintaining a healthy diet when eating out can be very challenging. The best way to do this is to plan before eating at a restaurant. As long as you set realistic expectations of yourself, commit, and reassess your progress, you can continue to follow the 1200 calorie diet plan.

Can I Drink Alcohol/Soda/Sweet Tea/Juice and Still Lose Weight?

Don't Drink Calories. When you eat the right amount of calories to lose weight, but when you drink alcohol, soda, sweet tea, juice, etc., those liquid calories count even though they don't fill you up. These calories either prevent you from losing weight or cause you to gain weight. What's worse is that the calories you drink have no effect on your hunger.

You don't even realize that you drink 250 calories during your meal, but if you drink a glass of water with zero calories, you do. If you want to lose weight, keep an eye on the drinks in your household as there may be high calorie drinks that can hinder your weight loss goals.

Those who think that fruit juice is good for our health are wrong because fruit juice is high in sugar content and also high in calories because fruit juices are not advertised as drinks but as a song they contain a lot of calories. If you think that diet drinks are better for your health than sugary drinks, they are not. According to researchers, diet drinks are lower in calories than sugary drinks, but they make you accustomed to the sweet taste. Studies have shown that after consuming the diet drinks regularly, the person Weight gain instead of weight loss.

Artificial sweeteners are also a problem. The sweetness of artificial sweeteners releases dopamine in the brain, which is the happiness hormone. This results in cravings for candy, ice cream, chocolate cake, and weight gain. They help but only if taken in small amounts.

Coffee is not high in calories. If you drink black coffee, it is good for your health because the caffeine in coffee in fact promotes fat burn. If you want to lose weight, you should cut down on your wine, beer, or champagne because the alcohol in them adds a lot of fat and calories to your body.

You should stay away from alcohol as it makes you more hungry as a result of which you gain weight. Ice cream and tea may seem low in calories, but they are high in sugar. A glass of tea contains 150 calories and 15 gram of sugar. The World Health Organization advises that adults consume no more than 25 grams of total sugar per day.

Do I have to drink milk to get calcium?

Dairy products such as milk cheese and yogurt are high in calcium, with about 250 to 350 milligrams per serving. Adults need 1,000 to 1200 milligrams of calcium per day. Dairy products are certainly an easy and convenient way to get the calcium your body needs, but they are not the only way. Fortified plant-based nuts, such as almonds, cashews, etc., contain about 300 milligrams of calcium per serving, as do canned salmon or sardines with bones. Broccoli has 40 milligrams per cup, and foods such as black almonds, white beans, and tofu have about a 100 milligrams of calcium per serving. Whether or not your diet includes dairy products, some careful planning can help you get enough calcium.

How to deal with hunger on diet?
Eating more protein in your diet can help you feel fuller for longer and consequently help you eat less at your next meal. According to the advice of researchers, we should eat protein equal to our body weight every day. Choose foods that are high in fiber. By slowing digestion, high fiber controls appetite so you feel full longer. Adding protein along with fiber can have double the benefits of reducing hunger.

Evidence suggests that drinking water can suppress appetite and lead to weight loss for some people. One study found that people who drank a glass of water before a meal ate 22 percent less food than those who didn't. Neurons are closely related. Choose solid foods to reduce hunger Two recent studies have found that solid foods reduce hunger significantly more than liquids. The solution is to focus on the food in front of you

Eat slowly It can be especially easy to eat more than you intended when you're very hungry. Slowing down the speed at which you eat can be one way to curb the tendency to overeat. According to researchers, people who eat fast eat more calories per day. Get regular exercise. Exercise reduces the activation of areas of the brain associated with food, which reduces the motivation to eat high-calorie foods.

How to avoid junk food?

Junk food is high in calories but low in nutrients. These foods are high in saturated fat and trans fat. Eating too much junk food can reduce eating healthy food. Also, eating more junk food increases potential risk of medical issues. Junk food like potato chips, cookies, candy, soda can give you momentarily happiness but not help you stay healthy. You need to adopt some good habits to avoid junk food.

Planning meals ahead of time reduces the amount of junk food you eat. Planning increases the amount of home-cooked meals in your daily diet. It also reduces the chances of craving for junk food. Make it a habit to eat foods rich in protein and good fats that will keep you feeling full longer and reduce cravings for junk food. Include fruits and vegetables in the diet as they are high in fiber. The fibers in these foods reduce food cravings.

Stop buying junk food because we are trying to avoid junk food. Buy healthy food only and buy food like fruits, vegetables, milk, eggs. Keep healthy food with you. It helps to keep junk food long. Drinking plenty of water keeps your body sugar balanced and makes you feel fuller longer. When you want to eat junk food, chewing sugar free mint gum will distract you and make whatever you eat taste weird.

Weight gain post dieting as the body attempts to regain equilibrium

Researchers say that the human body has a set point of weight. Even if you lose weight below the weight set point, the human body regains it back. If you start eating less, your body will gradually burn calories. Burn fewer calories even if your activity level doesn't change. Factors that can change your hormones and increase your appetite can make it easier for you to gain weight.

A set point is an idea because there is no real evidence. Researchers have observed that many people fall into a certain weight range, but weight is difficult to study scientifically. Just as your body helps you regain the weight you've lost, does it help you lose weight after you've gained it? Scientists have worked to answer the question: Is it easier to gain weight if we have a system that regulates body fat?

According to researchers, starvation has been the greatest threat to humans throughout history. Our bodies have evolved a way to protect us from starvation by holding on to fat. Obesity has only become a health hazard in recent years. Perhaps our bodies have not yet evolved to deal with obesity.

HOW TO KEEP THE WEIGHT LOSS
Even if the set point theory is right, it is possible to lose weight and keep it off. Avoid fad diets and sudden weight loss. You may need to lose weight slowly so your set point may change and your body may need to adjust to a new eating pattern. Taking the help of a dietitian can help you achieve success quickly.

How to avoid Nutrient deficiency on low-calorie diet?

People who eat restrictive diets are not getting all the nutrients their bodies need. People who choose low-carb diets to lose weight may be deficient in certain nutrients, including vitamin C, folate, magnesium, iron, vitamin B, and vitamin C. Calcium is a common nutrient that can be deficient.

Consider each micronutrient to ensure your body will function optimally on a low-carb diet. Then include nutritious foods in your meals throughout the day. Researchers have discovered that there are many nutrients in foods that we weren't aware of before or that need to work together in the foods we eat, in addition to the fact that supplements may not always provide the amount of nutrients we need, even if they say so on the label.

No matter how well we eat, our body is likely to be lacking some type of nutrient.

- Water: Dry skin, low energy, constipation.
- Vitamins and minerals: Low energy and poor immune function.
- Protein: This can happen when you are not eating enough protein-rich foods. Low amounts of lean muscle tissue, low energy, reduced strength, and not recovering from your workouts.
- Essential fatty acids: Poor immunity, inflammation, up and down blood sugar and reduced satiety.

Here are four ways to minimize nutritional deficiencies in your diet.

Focus on Protein
Animal-based foods such as meat, poultry, fish, eggs, and dairy products are good sources of protein. Black beans, lima beans, corn, salmon, broccoli are also good sources of protein.

Increase Hydration

Drink fluids before you feel thirsty. Use the color of your urine as an indicator to know if you are consuming enough fluids. If the color of your urine is pale yellow, fluid intake should be considered correct. If you see a dark yellow color, increase the intake.

ABOUT THE AUTHOR

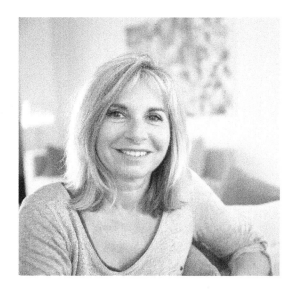

surgery to lose weight, and she lost over 100 pounds in just 3 months. She suffered great life changes after reaching 600 pounds, including becoming housebound, and, at times, feeling suicidal. Catharine decided to write a series of books on the "Now Diet" to make other people in the same situation feel motivated to take the path that led her to a new life.

Catharine Smith is the pseudonym of a patient of Dr. Nowzaradan. Catharine followed Dr. Nowzaradan's "Now Diet" days before her

Made in the USA
Las Vegas, NV
26 February 2023